May 13, 1984

Happy Mother's Day Grandma,

With much love,

Sharon

A VIEW
OF THE
MOUNTAINS

A VIEW
OF THE
MOUNTAINS

MORRIS GIBSON

BEAUFORT BOOKS, INC.
New York

*In the text the names and descriptions of characters have
been fictionalized except for those physicians and public
figures whose identities it would be impossible to conceal.*

*The poem, "The Hunters", p. 197, is reprinted by
kind permission of Florence B. Freedman.*

Library of Congress Cataloging in Publication Data

Gibson, Morris.
A view of the mountains.

Sequel to: One man's medicine.
1. Gibson, Morris. 2. Physicians (General practice) —
Great Britain — Biography. 3. Physicians (General
practice) — Canada — Biography. I. Title.
R489.G48A38 1983   610'.92'4 [B]   83-19728
ISBN 0-8253-0186-6

Published in the United States by Beaufort Books, Inc., New York.
Published in Canada by Collins Publishers, Toronto

Printed in the U.S.A.   First American Edition

10 9 8 7 6 5 4 3 2 1

To Janet
With Love

ACKNOWLEDGEMENTS

I wish to express my acknowledgements to Fred and Helen Wooding for their help and advice, to James and Helen Herriot for their warm encouragement, and to Squadron Leader Cy Goodwin for his kindness in typing the manuscript and keeping my infinitives "on course"; to Janet for her patience and to many old friends and patients who have given me permission to write about themselves or close relatives.

Prologue

"So you're emigrating, Gibson. And to Canada?"

"That's right."

"Toronto?"

"No."

"Montreal, then. An interesting city," said my colleague reflectively. "The meeting place of two great cultures. A sophisticated sort of place, I should think."

"We're not going to Montreal."

"Oh! Ah, Vancouver, of course! It's a beautiful city, they tell me – mountains, the sea, and all that kind of thing."

My inquisitor warmed his well-tailored bottom before the fireplace in Quern House, our medical club in Hull, Yorkshire. He was a specialist, a few years older than myself, and dressed in fashionable tweeds, he adopted an air of complacent benevolence as he spoke. He was rocking backward and forward a little on his heels. It was a well-practised little mannerism of his, and was calculated, I thought, to impress. He was slowly twirling the stem of his sherry glass between the forefinger and thumb of his right hand. His left hand was thrust into his jacket pocket.

"You'll like Vancouver," he beamed at me. "It'll be a bit of a change, of course, from the North Sea to the Pacific, but . . ."

"We're not going to Vancouver, either."

I hadn't meant to be curt or discourteous. I was preoccupied. I had resigned from Britain's National Health Service a week or so before. My bridges were burnt behind me, and the enormity of the step I was about to make my little family take weighed heavily upon me.

"Not Vancouver?"

Behind my colleague's spectacles the benign gaze had been replaced by one of deep concern. He carefully placed his sherry glass on the mantelpiece before he spoke again. He stood quite still, was silent for a moment, then exclaimed,

"Good God! Where *are* you going?"

I had dropped in at our club for lunch. Several doctors met there regularly, exchanged the medical gossip of the day and had a sherry or perhaps a beer before a light meal.

It was early March, 1955. The late winter gale drove the rain in sheets along the pavement. A passer-by hurried along, umbrella held tight and low against the force of the wind; a rivulet of rainwater snaked its way down the windowpane and cascaded from the sill to the pavement below. In the silence that followed his question, I could hear the rain splashing against the wall as it fell.

"We're going to a little cowtown in the foothills of the Rockies. Okotoks. It's about twenty-five miles south of Calgary in Alberta. They need a doctor and don't have one."

"Calgary! Alberta! I say, old boy, you must be joking! You *can't* go there! It's just not your kind of thing. It won't work. There's nothing there – no culture, no character. *Nobody* to talk to. Nothing but oil wells and gum-chewing cowboy types."

We were the only members to attend for lunch that day and so we abandoned the dining table and sought the solace of the fireplace. We were ensconced in comfortable chairs, our luncheon plates balanced on our knees, when my acquaintance spoke again.

"What on earth made you do it, old boy? It's not money, I know. You've got a very good practice. You've just bought that house out at West Ella, a beautiful spot too, so I'm told. So what in the name of heaven makes a man like you pull up stakes and take his wife and daughter to some God-forsaken spot on the Canadian prairies? What d'you call it again?"

"Okotoks. The population is six hundred and seventy if you want to know, with scattered ranches and farms in the surrounding countryside."

"Okotoks? It sounds like hell to me. Have you ever been to Western Canada?"

"No. I've been to Eastern Canada but never further west than Ontario."

"How far's Ontario from your precious Okotoks?"

"About two thousand miles."

"My God. Why don't you go to Turkey? It isn't any further away from civilization, if it's a change of scenery you're looking for!"

"I don't need any change of scenery," I replied. "I love it here, and until four or five years ago, I loved my work too. But

I'm not going to spend the rest of my life signing endless sick certificates and doing slaphappy, hurried medicine."

"What does Janet say to all this?"

"A couple of months ago, she said she'd be damned if she'd emigrate. But she's as frustrated as I am, and for a girl who used to speak at meetings in favor of a Health Service, that should say something!"

"What about Catriona?"

"Our little one is very secure. She's seen a bit of the States and Canada. It's a great adventure for her. My one promise is that she'll have her own pony, and not just one hired from the riding school!"

My companion turned his attention to his lunch for a few minutes, but I knew he was watching me.

"Tell me," he said, "what brought it to a head? And how did you choose this cowtown of yours?"

"For two years now, I've quietly been studying law. I'm nearly half way to being a lawyer and there have been many times when I've thought of getting out of medicine altogether. But we made our decision a few months ago. One night I'd been called out by a midwife who was having problems with one of her cases. I was out for an hour or two. We ended up with a forceps delivery and a few problems. When I got home, it was early morning and my brain was just racing, so I set the card table up by the fire – it was still smoldering – and I worked away at the Law of Torts and Contracts. I don't know how long I'd been there when I realized I wasn't alone. I turned round and there was Janet, curled up in a chair watching me. It was almost dawn."

"Darling," she said, "you'll get that law degree – but you'll never be anything but a doctor. We're going to emigrate."

"How on earth did you choose Okotoks?"

I smiled. "We were in the States a year ago, visiting an old buddy of mine in the U.S. Army. A wonderful old surgeon offered me a job in Washington, D.C., but I told him that if I emigrated I'd go where the Union Jack still flies."

"That was a bit touchy with an American, wasn't it?"

"Not at all. He'd worked as a medical missionary all over the world, and he told me there was still a frontier spirit in Western Canada. He said there were little towns in the foothills of the

Rockies that needed doctors. When we contacted the Canadian Immigration people, Janet and I had stipulated that we wanted to go where we were needed, not to a large city. We studied maps for hours and talked for days. The immigration people had given us the names of three towns in Alberta that needed doctors. One place seemed much the same as another."

Finally Janet said, "Let's make it Okotoks. It's got two OKs in it, so it's OK with me."

After lunch my colleague, doubtfully, wished me good luck.

The next few weeks were hectic. Preparations had to be made for our departure, relatives visited, our house at West Ella – Janet's dream home – sold. Catriona held little parties for her school friends. The three of us visited the school together to say goodbye to the teachers, to her beloved Miss Brooks and Miss Jefferson, the Head.

It was she who said to me, "I hope you realize, doctor, that you are taking from us the future Captain of the school."

To be Captain of Tranby meant something in East Yorkshire; the school had an excellent reputation and our little one had been happy there. But Catriona would soon enter a different world at the Okotoks High School.

The only time that tears were shed was when we took Prince, our faithful collie, to his new home. He could not travel with us.

Finally, with all our preparations for departure completed, we found time to take a holiday. It was a holiday with a purpose. Whatever the new world held in store for us, there was a heritage to remember, especially for our little one.

We went to London, visited the great art galleries, saw the Tower, toured Westminster Abbey, St. Paul's Cathedral and the Houses of Parliament. We traveled to Oxford, strolled round quiet quadrangles, and looked into dark corners at cold, austere little rooms where young men, destined to become great, had once studied.

We traveled to Scotland to see relatives and friends, stood by the shores of quiet lochs and wandered through deserted castles, their stone walls crumbling now, reminders of Scotland's often brutal past. But we visited our old University too, and talked of Scotland's place in science and medicine. Then it was back to Hull for that final week of cocktail parties and quiet dinners.

Our friends, medical and otherwise, reacted in various ways to our going. Some were envious; some encouraged us; some vowed to follow us – and several did. Some were sad and some indignant.

"Why," they said, "should you choose to leave the country when people like you are needed?"

It was at a cocktail party that someone said,

"What kind of job are you going out to?"

Before I could think of an appropriate reply, Janet had said, "We're not going out to any *job*. We're going to a little town that says it needs a doctor. We're not going out to some salaried appointment. We're just going to put our names up and hope that people will come to us. In fact," she finished emphatically, "we're going to have to *sell* ourselves."

"Janet," I interjected, "*I* may have to sell myself – but *you*? – *never*!"

Chapter
One

Janet and I had qualified as doctors in 1939 just at the outbreak of war. I joined the army within a few months while Janet, a classmate at the University of Glasgow Medical School, took up hospital work. We had married in 1941 and Catriona was born in 1943.

We had practised medicine in Hull – or, to give it its ancient and proper name, the City and County of Kingston-upon-Hull, in Yorkshire's ancient East Riding – since the end of the war. We were both general practitioners, although until the advent of the National Health Service in 1948, Janet had also been a sessional anesthetist at Hull's Women's Hospital. For eight years we had lived in the old house on Anlaby Road next door to our "surgery" or office, but in 1954 we had left our old, four-storeyed city home with all its drafts and dark corners, and moved to a modern house in West Ella, a lovely old village a few miles from our practice. We no longer had daily help. It was a small price to pay for privacy, said Janet whose work had been eased by Dr. Gilbert Swanson, another Scot, joining the practice.

Hull has a long history. In the twelfth century it was well known as a "wool port" and it still exports more wool than any other seaport in England. By the middle of the fourteenth century it was a walled and fortified town, and the king had granted it the right to hold markets. That open air market continues today much as it did centuries ago.

The city also has a long tradition of non-conformist independence. In the Civil War of the seventeenth century, the citizens refused to support the king in his struggle against Parliament. They defied King Charles. Twice the aldermen closed the city gates against his army and eventually the Royalists rode away. That spirit of defiance lived on during the Second World War, as over the years Hull suffered more damage and sustained more casualties than Coventry.

The medical community was a friendly one. The hospitals had excellent reputations and were able to attract highly qualified

1

doctors to work in them, yet there was none of the anonymity that inevitably develops when cities become very large. Many of us, general practitioners and specialists alike, were on first name terms with one another.

Perhaps we owed some of that informal friendliness to the use we made of our medical club, a comfortable old house near the center of town. It had a lecture hall and facilities for small groups to meet over drinks or a meal. Lectures, often by eminent specialists from London, were given regularly and were well attended. At the conclusion of such lectures we might meet in the dining room for port or a parting whisky.

They were not always solemn occasions. One distinguished visitor gave a very undistinguished lecture on spinal meningitis. He delivered his message in a monotone and I could see some of his listeners were indulging in quiet naps throughout the talk. At the end of his lecture, however, and after a whisky, he became very voluble.

It turned out that his greatest interest was not so much in his own specialty as in psychoanalysis. He was an enthusiast. He had, he said euphorically to one of our psychiatrists, undergone a seven-year course of psychoanalysis by one of London's leading analysts, and "do you know," he announced with evangelical zeal, "at the end of it I was a changed man."

He had found a soulmate in the psychiatrist. The two left the room together, deep in conversation, presumably to continue the discussion elsewhere. There was a sudden silence. The change in the man, from dull lecturer to vociferous champion of psychoanalysis had been startling.

Then one of my colleagues whose cultured accent, dignified demeanor, fancy waistcoats and hussar's moustache hid a sharp and irreverent wit, drawled thoughtfully,

"I say, you fellows! About this psychoanalysis thing. Do you think the old boy was daft before – or after?"

But more than the medical society met at the club. The Syndicate, as we were dubbed, met there. I had been instrumental in forming the Syndicate. Prior to the war, "single-handed" practitioners had outnumbered doctors working in groups in Britain.

2

In 1946, after demobilization, I had persuaded a neighboring doctor that we would benefit from "standing in" for one another on alternate nights and weekends. The only exception was for obstetrics. We would deliver our own babies. Within six months there were six of us in the group. We all remained in independent practice but for ten years, not a night call went unanswered and not a penny changed hands. We arranged coverage for holidays and in cases of illness. We became friends as much as colleagues. Our wives became acquainted. We held dinner parties among ourselves and were the envy of less fortunate colleagues. Potential recruits were advised to form their own emergency groups, for, we said, too many physicians would spoil the emergency service. The groups had to be compact entities and serve compact areas.

We met monthly in the clubhouse when we would arrange the duty roster and hold formal clinical meetings. At 10 p.m. precisely we closed the educational sessions and opened the bar. Not that we overindulged, but it is the case that for years the Hull Medical Society, chronically short of funds, facetiously but with due ceremony passed an annual vote of thanks to the Syndicate for its generous financial support!

Now it was the spring of 1955. On this particular morning, I had been enroute from one house call to another and had decided to stop my car to get a breath of fresh air.

The fast waters of the Humber River were deceptively smooth, I thought, as I leaned against the railings of Prince's Pier and gazed across the estuary.

There had been a fog earlier but the sun was beginning to shine through and only a haze remained. I could see the low outlines of the Lincolnshire shore a mile or two away on the south side of the estuary. Behind me lay the city of Hull. Behind me, too, I could hear the bustle of dockside activity, the engines of ships' cranes at work, trucks being maneuvered and directions shouted as cargo was moved. There was a salty tang in the air together with that familiar dockside amalgam of fruity smells from the warehouses, hot diesel oil, tar and gasoline. One of my quiet pleasures was to watch the dockside scene as I was doing now and I should have been enjoying myself.

I wasn't. My right index finger, swathed in bandages, was aching and throbbing mercilessly.

A year or two previously I had on impulse invested our entire savings in a pig farm. It seemed to me at the time to be a brilliant move. Janet's opinion, when she learned of my investment, was less favorable. My pig farming activities were seldom the subject of light-hearted breakfast conversation.

Yesterday a pig had bitten me. My associate had phoned to say that one of the piglets was ill and that my medical advice would be welcomed. I draw this distinction between my wife and partner, and my associate. My associate was the chap with whom I had gone into the pig business. I answered his call, for my main contribution to the association (apart, of course, from our entire savings) was my knowledge of medicine and its application to piggy ailments.

That piglet was indeed ill. I didn't have the slightest idea of what was causing the trouble. It was, I thought, some acute infection and so I suggested the blunderbuss treatment of an injection of penicillin into muscle, plus getting the animal to swallow a tablet or two of sulphonamide.

The injection was easy. So was the first tablet. My associate held the piglet's mouth open while I popped the tablet onto the back of its tongue. It was the second tablet that proved my undoing. Pigs, even little ones, are surprisingly perceptive creatures, and the sight of that second tablet was enough to set off a chorus of squealing, struggling objections. Full of confidence in my ability, I had neglected to use the little funnel down which one can slide a pill. My associate's grip slipped at the crucial moment and piggy jaws clamped shut with my right index finger between them. I could feel the teeth crunch on the bone. However, my finger remained intact.

It was not a happy experience and I had taken myself off to the Western General Hospital. Dr. John Coates, the senior surgeon and a friend of mine, had just finished an emergency operation when I arrived. It seemed to me that considering the gravity of my wound, there was a good deal of hilarity from the operating room staff at my explanation of how I had been injured, but I was invited to make myself comfortable on the operating-room table, while the wound was attended to.

4

"It should be all right," said John, when he had finished and had given me a tetanus booster injection. "But in any case I'll see you tomorrow night at the Hull Medical Society meeting. I'm lecturing on abnormalities of the lower bowel, if you remember."

"Thanks very much, John," I had said, "I'll be there."

That next morning on the pier I was feeling the aftereffects of my injury. However, I was refreshed by my stroll around the docks. I had lunch and waded through the evening office session, a long and tedious one, before I headed for the medical clubhouse and John's lecture.

It was in progress when I arrived. There were fifty or sixty doctors present and quietly I slipped in by the back door of the lecture room. But not quietly enough.

Dr. Coates looked up from his notes, paused and called out, "Just one moment, Gibson, please. Would you mind standing just where you are?"

Every head was turned in my direction. Embarrassed, I stood rooted to the spot. John was the best natured of fellows, but obviously I had disturbed his lecture and must pay the price for my interruption. Heads were turned toward the lecturer again and as I stood there trying to look inconspicuous, he continued.

"It is always advisable, gentlemen, that in any physical examination you should carry out a rectal examination. That exploring finger inside the anus is of inestimable value.

"And now," he declaimed, "Gibson – would you step forward and hold up your right hand so that we can all see it?"

The cynosure of all eyes, I held my hand on high. That bandaged finger stood out like a lighthouse.

"You see," said Dr. Coates, with a grin, "Gibson *always* does rectal examinations!"

Chapter Two

We had visited America in the spring of 1954. Dr. Christensen, who had befriended me in Washington D.C., said as we shook hands for the last time before we made for New York, the old *Queen Mary* and home, "You'll be back. I'll give you a year."

His remark haunted me and in that summer of 1954, I found my restlessness returning. And yet how I loved my friends "at home" and how I loved to wander in the dales of the East Riding. And how difficult it was going to be for me to take a step that would be irrevocable – emigration.

Perhaps that is why I cherish my memories of the dales that year.

Exercise in the fresh air is an important part of life and it is easy to get in East Yorkshire where the winds from the North Sea blow across the plain toward the dales.

There are excellent golf courses and tennis clubs, but my friend Ernie Denton and I enjoyed simpler pleasures. We went for long walks together. Sometimes we might hike along the cliffs overlooking the sea or on country roads where we could see the broad plain, but we were drawn more to the Humber foreshore and to East Yorkshire's dales. They lack the wind-swept bareness of the moors further north. They are smaller, more intimate places, sheltered, well treed, and a joy for the hiker.

Not that Ernest and I hiked. We never had set goals or deadlines. We tramped, and causally at that. With his ready wit and cheery smile, Ernie, a bluff Yorkshireman of about my own age who had been a navigator in wartime with the RAF Bomber Force, was an ideal companion, and for years we tramped the dales together in our spare time. In summer we might lounge on some hillside and bask in the sun, watching coasters beat their way up the estuary, their bow waves white against the patchy blues and greys of the river. In the winter cold we kept moving, striding briskly along.

We got to know some of the dales' farmers who suggested that we might shoot over their land, which was infested with rabbits. British wild rabbits made excellent eating, as many wartime diners who had eaten chicken à la king in London restaurants could confirm. However, we stopped bringing rabbits home. They were neither welcomed nor appreciated by our wives. The trouble was – they were flea-infested. Having once been forbidden the pleasures of the connubial couch until I had undressed, hung my clothes in the open air, and led any surviving fleas to a watery grave in the bath, I decided against this free source of protein, however appealing to my Scottish instincts!

When summer became fall, with the cold winds sweeping in from the sea, we no longer lingered on our walks, although one of our continuing pleasures was a glass of beer at the end of an outing.

It was in Bill Siggle's kitchen one afternoon having a beer that I realized we had a very unusual host. Bill was a farmer, and we were always welcomed in his old, low-ceilinged farmhouse, where the roof beams were black and gnarled with age, the stone floor worn concave in places from the passage of hobnailed boots over the generations.

Bill had left us for a few minutes, when Ernie, who had been idly looking out of the kitchen window, suddenly exclaimed,

"Cor-blimey, doc, come and look at this!"

Waddling across the farmyard was a gargoyle of a duck. It was like no duck I had ever seen. Its short legs seemed barely able to support its fat, round body topped by a head that surely belonged to a turkey. We watched it, intrigued, unaware that Siggles, tankard in hand, had walked up behind us and was also watching the animal.

"Gee," said Ernie, "I've never seen anything as ugly as that in my life – beggin' your pardon, Bill," he added hastily, realizing that our host stood beside us.

But Bill Siggles wasn't put out. He seemed pleased that we had taken notice of the creature.

"Don't worry lad," he assured Ernie. "No apology's needed. But I will agree 'e's an ugly owd sinner. But you know, doctor,

7

that yonder is an interesting case for *you* to study – you bein'
a man of science."

"Oh?"

"Aye. It's not every day you'll see the likes of 'im. You see,
I'm a bit of an experimenter myself. Now, I know nowt about
science, y' understand – but that bird is the result of one of my
experiments. I'd just about given up hope of getting results –
but there 'e is – a cross between a turkey and a duck."

With suddenly awakened interest, I watched the creature as
it waddled towards a low step at the barn door, hopped on to
it and disappeared inside the building.

I turned to our host. He was sipping his beer. With his burly
build, dressed in old tweeds, knee-high rubber boots and a cloth
cap perched precariously on the back of his head, he did not
look like a man with innate scientific talents.

"Amazing," I said.

"Aye," replied Mr. Siggles, "I thought ye'd be interested."

"Interested? I'm intrigued. But this should be published in a
scientific journal . . . "

Siggles interrupted me.

"No, no," he told me with typical Yorkshire reticence. "It's
nowt to boast about. I just get me own pleasure out o't."

He wouldn't be budged. But on our way home Ernest and I
discussed the experiment. It shouldn't be left at that, we said.
Somebody should be told. It was the subject of conversation for
some time, and I brought it up to an interested audience at a
small academic dinner at the University College; but with the
winter came an epidemic of respiratory infections. The practice
work was overwhelming and Siggles' experiment forgotten.

Christmas was near and we hadn't seen our beloved dales for
weeks when one Saturday morning, in Whitefriargate, I met Bill
Siggles.

I would have passed him by, failing to recognize him, well
dressed in business suit, trilby hat and heavy overcoat, but he
hailed me. Bill wasn't just a simple farmer, I had learned. He
was a successful one and a prosperous man despite the appearance created when wearing work clothes.

"Doctor, I 'aven't seen you two lads for weeks. What 'ave
ye been up to?"

"Just busy, Bill – too much sickness to get a day off."

"Aye – well doan't be too busy next Saturday. An' tell Ernie, will ye? I 'ave a bird for each of ye for Christmas. So come down for lunch and we'll 'ave a glass of ale beforehand."

And he was off, on his way to see his accountant in Hull's Land of Green Ginger, a little lane that has seen the centuries go by, and still remains part of the city's business district.

Saturday soon came round. It was a gloomy day. The rain was pouring as Ernie and I set off in my car. As we splashed our way along I thought my crony was unusually silent.

"It's just," said Ernie, in response to my query, "that I like Bill Siggles, but if he tries to pawn that bloody experiment of his on to me, I'll have to offend him. I'm not going to take it. I could never face fowl again." He lapsed into silence.

"Mind you," he said, a mile or two further on, "it's good of Bill to think of us – but there *are* limits, doc, you will agree?"

I agreed, but pointed out that after all, the flesh of fowl is acceptable and many fish that have a most unattractive appearance are considered delicacies. Ernest was not reassured.

We arrived at the farmhouse and tramped into the kitchen. A bright fire roared in the huge fireplace. The whitewashed ceiling reflected the flames and even its black beams added to the warmth of the place; the festive appearance of the room was completed by cases of beer and bottles of liquor on a side table.

The wooden kitchen table was loaded with birds, dozens of them, all cleaned and dressed. The only somber note was the one picture that graced the wall. It was a print of a gloomy Napoleon, leading his army on the retreat from Moscow. The symbolism of this was not then apparent to me.

"Well, lads," said Bill, "I've got summat I must do for a few minutes. Just help yourselves to t'drinks," and he left us alone.

In an instant Ernest reached the table. A whirlwind seemed to hit it. Birds were picked up, inspected and thrown aside. Finally he returned to his chair. Instantly he had become my bluff and hearty companion again.

"It isn't there," he whispered. "I'd know it anywhere!"

He raised his tankard and with great gusto wished me a merry Xmas.

9

At that very moment I looked out of the window.

"There it is, Ernie," I cried.

Sure enough, our friend was waddling across the farmyard. We were watching it, fascinated, when our host returned and joined us at the window.

"Aye," he chuckled. " 'E's an ugly owd son of a gun. But ye know," he added, "I wouldn't be wi'out 'im for all t'tea in China – t'owd Muscovy duck."

"Muscovy duck?" I cried.

"Aye, that's 'im. I still mind the day I bought 'im."

"Bought him?"

Our host was oblivious of my startled responses.

" 'E's wot's called an exotic species. 'E's got nowt t'do wi' Moscow. 'E's from the joongles of the Amazon, so they tell me, an' why the 'ell they call 'im a Muscovy duck is beyond me.

"Aye, but I 'ave t' tell ye lads," he went on conspiratorially, "I've 'ad some fun wi' 'im in my time. Ye know, every silly city bugger as comes 'ere I tell 'em it's a cross between a turkey and a duck – and lads, ye'd hardly credit it, but they all believe me."

"Ernie!" he cried in alarm. "What's matter, lad? It's not like thee to choke on thy ale!"

Chapter Three

That last year in England was not to be without its drama.

By four o'clock one afternoon, I had finished the day's house calls with two hours to go before the evening surgery. I'd headed home for a relaxing cup of tea.

Janet met me at the door.

"There's someone waiting in the sitting room," she said. "He's a very nice man and says he must talk to us."

"What's someone doing sitting in our front room at this time in the afternoon?" I asked a little peevishly. "And what does he do for a living that he can spend afternoons sitting around?"

"He's a police officer," replied Janet sweetly, "a detective inspector."

"Oh! Did he say what he wanted?" I asked, somewhat taken aback.

"No – just that he has to talk to us."

"What's his name?"

"Detective Inspector Lumsden."

"Never heard of him. Let's see what he wants."

Our visitor, who was sitting by the fire, rose as we entered the room, came forward and shook hands. He wasn't a tall man for a policeman and in his neat grey suit he wouldn't have been conspicuous in any crowd; but he was friendly and had an openness of expression that made me trust him at first sight. He was in his late forties, I judged, grey-haired, slim and courteous.

"D' you mind if I smoke?" he asked.

He proffered his own cigarette case. Janet, having met a soulmate, accepted a cigarette and lit it with practised skill. Then our visitor spoke.

"Do you people know Edward John Briggs?"

"Yes," replied Janet. "He and his wife are patients of ours."

The inspector nodded.

"That's our information. We also understand that Mrs. Briggs has been treated for high blood pressure. Is that correct?"

Janet, who obviously liked our visitor, made it clear, however, that she wasn't inclined to discuss her patient's condition casually. The police officer reassured her.

"This is official. Mrs. Briggs won't be coming back to you. She's dead. She died following an assault by her husband. He's in jail, charged with manslaughter and is to stand trial at York Assizes on March fifteenth next."

"Inspector," I said, "this is news to us. It must have happened while we were on holiday. But how are we involved?"

"Our information," said the detective, "is that Mrs. Biggs had very high blood pressure for years."

"Correct."

11

"Was it high enough that a sudden fall or even excitement could have brought on a stroke?"

"It's possible," replied Janet.

The detective turned to me.

"Do you agree with your wife's opinion?"

"Yes, I do," I replied.

The treatment of "hypertension" has been revolutionized in the last thirty years, but at that time, effective drugs were few. Janet went on to explain the mechanism of cerebral hemorrhage. The inspector busied himself with his notebook, nodded when Janet finished, and said,

"In other words, it needn't have been a blow that killed her? Quite independently she could have had a stroke, just at the very moment her husband struck her?"

"Inspector, could you explain what this is all about before we go any further?"

"I'm sorry," replied our visitor, "but could I ask a few more questions first? Tell me, did Briggs seem to you to be a violent man?"

Indeed, he never had. He was a rather pathetic figure, a man in his fifties who seldom smiled; short, overweight, plethoric. He had been born in a dark little house in one of those alleys that littered the poorer parts of the city, and he had lived there all his life, an unskilled laborer, like his father before him.

"That's about right," said Mr. Lumsden when I finished. "You see, we know a bit about Briggs and his wife – from neighbors and the policeman on the beat. Witnesses will testify that they quarreled – right on their front doorstep; that Briggs struck his wife and that she fell. She became unconscious and died two days later. There's some conflicting evidence as to whether he kicked or hit her a second time. But that was that and Briggs was duly charged with manslaughter."

"It sounds very straightforward," I remarked.

The inspector looked at me unsmilingly.

"Perhaps there's more to it than just the obvious facts," he said.

"And there usually is," added Janet tersely.

The inspector continued,

"Briggs has never been in trouble with the police, was never

12

known to beat his wife. The neighbors say they were a quiet couple who kept to themselves. I think it says a bit that when we went through the house, everything was in perfect order – dishes clean, pots shining, beds well made.

"But you know, with hard times come pressures and anger – and Briggs lost his job six months ago. He's been drinking – never been known to do that either. And his wife maybe just didn't know how to handle him, so she started nagging him; sometimes in front of the neighbors. And that's when it all happened. Maybe Briggs just expressed his anger the only way he knew how – he struck out. Oh! It wasn't any accident," he went on, "he struck her all right."

"So, inspector, where do we come in?"

"The whole case has bothered me," he replied, "and I've been turning it over in my mind. They did a post-mortem examination. Now there was no bruising around the scalp or face consistent with a blow. There was no fracture of the skull. What there was, though, was a massive cerebral hemorrhage, and the pathologist said there was extensive atherosclerosis – that's hardening of the arteries, isn't it?"

"Generally speaking, yes."

"When I heard about her high blood pressure, I put two and two together. You people were her family doctors, so here I am. Was her blood pressure high enough, that taken in conjunction with the unhealthy state of her arteries, she could have had a fatal stroke just with excitement – a quarrel, being hit, not even forcibly enough to do damage?"

"It's an interesting theory!"

"Is it a possibility?"

"Yes," we both said in unison.

"Then," said the police officer, "would one of you appear in court and say so?"

"Inspector Lumsden," I said, astonished, "you're asking us to give evidence that could damage, even destroy your own case?"

"Possibly," he replied, his face expressionless.

"Evidence for the defence, in fact?"

"No sir. It would be evidence for us – for the prosecution,

13

the police. We'd see you get all the correct papers. Will you do it?"

"Yes," said Janet, "we must. My husband will do it. He's made more court appearances than I," she added with a smile.

I had one final word.

"You're an unusual policeman. It was pretty good thinking on your part and it's pretty humane to take this interest in the man."

"I don't know about that," replied Mr. Lumsden. "You doctors are jealous of *your* reputations – most of you, that is!" he added with a half smile. "So are we coppers – most of us. I'd hate to see a man go to jail if there's a reasonable doubt about his guilt.

"But, I warn you, His Lordship is a hard man to convince. It won't be enough to produce character witnesses to say Briggs is a decent chap who didn't really mean any harm. The medical evidence'll be vital. Give your opinion firmly. The judge may listen. If he doesn't – believe me – Briggs is in real trouble."

He shook hands with us at the front door.

"Till the Assizes then," he said as he took his leave.

The Courts of Assize are a constant reminder of the history, the majesty of the English Common Law.

Scots Law, strangely enough, is based on Roman Law, yet the Romans never conquered Scotland. They occupied parts of it from time to time. Perhaps they thought my homeland, with its mists and rain, wasn't worth the trouble of conquest. But they occupied England for centuries, and although their roads remain, serviceable still in places, their Law has all but vanished.

The English Common Law is the child of later inhabitants. The Courts of Assize were founded some time in the twelfth century by that great king, Henry II, in order to bring "the King's peace" to all parts of his realm. At those Courts of Assize the King's judges meted out the King's justice. The Justices of Assize were itinerant or circuit judges and after nearly eight centuries, those same circuits remain.

In his reforms, Henry abolished trials by ordeal and combat. He made certain crimes offences not against the individual, but against the Crown, thus laying the foundation for England's system of Law. To cause a person's death was such an offence, and under those rules of law, founded eight centuries before, Edward John Briggs had been called to account.

The Justices of Assize still travel the length and breadth of England dispensing the law, and in some cases making it, for the *obiter dicta* – the "sayings by the way" of the great judges, the legal precedents they set in their judgments – have often molded the judicial system. It is not a perfect instrument, for Justice is not necessarily synonymous with the Law. But the Common Law of England, with its ability to adapt and expand to meet the juridical needs of the changing centuries, lives on, a treasure in our democratic heritage.

Those thoughts were in my mind that March 15 as I stood with the gowned and wigged barristers, with policemen and spectators, waiting for the trumpeters to announce – as they have done for centuries – the arrival of the Justices of Assize. On arrival they would move in solemn procession to those austere courtrooms that have seen so much of drama and tragedy.

I had waited like this before. The unchanging ceremony, the sense of "occasion" has always left me with a feeling of history, of the strength of human society.

I had always had an interest in the law, not so much in the day-to-day matters that must concern every lawyer, but more academically perhaps, in the history and development of law, especially the English Common Law, over the centuries. The Briggs case was to be heard before one of the great courts of England, and I'd been particularly intrigued by the attitude of the enlightened and humane policeman, Lumsden. He seemed to me to be the embodiment of good law, which guards our liberties and speaks for the moral sentiments of a people. But how would Briggs fare? Would the court merely interpret the rules of law – or would it see justice done?

Suddenly, as we stood there in the cold morning breeze, there was movement in the waiting crowd, a policeman hurried past, and just as my companion, counsel for the prosecution in the Briggs case, said, "I think they've arrived," the trumpets shrilled their summons. The icy high notes cut through the morning air, rising and reverberating before their echoes ebbed and died away.

However, my feelings of awe speedily dissolved into quiet laughter when the heralds appeared, dressed in their medieval tabards, leading the justices. The heralds were two tiny elderly men.

"These little men," I whispered, "and what a noise they made. It might have been the Archangel Gabriel himself."

Counsel did not answer my smile.

"Laugh now, my friend," he murmured, "there will be precious little laughing when His Lordship has finished this session. And those trumpets may well have sounded the knell of doom for someone."

The judge who would try the Briggs case led the procession. Silent, my companion bowed from the waist as His Lordship in the grey wig, black gown and scarlet sash of high office, oblivious of the policemen standing at rigid attention or the bows of barristers, stepped silently by, stony-faced and ominous.

The first case to be heard was one of attempted murder. Timothy Horton, heavily handsome and well dressed, didn't look the kind of man who would brutally batter his wife, leave her lying on the kitchen floor, cold-bloodedly borrow a cudgel from a neighbor, return and attempt to kill her. But the evidence was incontrovertible. Neighbors, hearing the woman's screams, had summoned the police who arrested Horton in the act of beating his wife about the head. She had spent many months in hospital recovering from serious injuries.

The evidence given, the jury retired briefly. The verdict – "guilty."

Having asked the prisoner if he had anything to say, His Lordship pronounced sentence. His voice was calm, coldly courteous.

"You, Timothy Horton, having committed a dastardly and cowardly assault, with intent to kill, will be taken to one of Her Majesty's prisons, there to spend ten years at hard labor."

Suddenly there was a scream. Horton's wife sitting in court called to the judge,

"Oh, Your Lordship, have mercy. It was all my fault. I drove him to it. I forgive him."

The judge was making notes and looked up from his writing.

16

"Madam," he said politely, "the crime was not yours to for-give. Society cannot condone such premeditated brutality."

In two sentences he had summed up the functions of today's Courts of Assize. From the sole medieval authority of the King, the courts have progressed to meet the demands of society, although the procedure of trial has changed little over the ages. Horton's crime was against society, and society, vested in the symbol of the Crown, had tried him.

The drama, however, was not quite over. In her agony of mind Mrs. Horton screamed again, pleading for mercy for her husband.

His Lordship hardly looked up from his notes.

"Take that woman away," he said.

With that quiet, cultured voice of his, he might have been the Archbishop of Canterbury pronouncing a benediction.

As we filed out for lunch I spoke to one of the detectives from Hull.

"Phew!" I exclaimed. "That judge puts the fear of God in me!"

"You're right," grunted my acquaintance. "I've seen him sentence men to the gallows and show less emotion."

"What's going to happen to Briggs this afternoon?"

"Search me, doc – but believe me, your evidence had better be good."

Somehow I didn't need lunch that day. I just wanted to get away from that place.

In courts of law, medical evidence is almost always useful, and in cases like the Briggs affair it can be crucial. It must also be exact, supported by accurate notes and records, and it must be unprejudiced. The ill-prepared medical witness can speedily find himself at the mercy of acid-tongued counsel for one side or the other, and treated with veiled contempt by judges.

But, I told myself, counsel for Briggs' defence wasn't going to challenge me and the lawyer for the prosecution might even prompt me if I didn't make my remarks succinctly enough.

When the court reassembled, Edward John Briggs, looking older and thinner than I remembered him, took his place in the

17

dock. I retired to the room reserved for witnesses. One by one we were called to the stand. The afternoon dragged on while my apprehension increased. Finally my turn came.

After being sworn in, I described the severity of Mrs. Briggs' hypertension, stating under questioning that she could have had a stroke at any time, and that, in the absence of any damage to the skull, or even bruising, it was conceivable that she had in fact gone into irreversible coma, not as the result of any blow, but because of a sudden stroke.

A few perfunctory questions were asked by both counsel. My task was over. I was about to leave the stand when His Lordship leaned forward and spoke in that controlled voice.

"One moment, doctor, if you please."

It was that icy courtesy of his that disturbed me.

"Here it comes," I said to myself. "Just keep cool, old boy."

"Your evidence makes it clear, doctor, does it not, that in your opinion, it is conceivable that the accused's wife may have died, not as the result of violence, but as the result of physical illness?"

"Yes, my lord, that is my belief."

"And you have sound medical grounds for this opinion?"

"Yes, my lord."

"In other words, there is, in your opinion, reasonable doubt as to the cause of death?"

"Yes, my lord."

"Thank you. You may go."

Sweating quietly, I did that, but I slipped back into court to hear the judge's final remarks to the jury.

Briggs had unquestionably struck his wife, said His Lordship. She had fallen to the ground and had become unconscious, dying two days later. "At the same time . . ." and out came my opinion. The judge finished. The jury, he said, must retire and consider their verdict.

The court was called to order. His Lordship retired. The jury filed out and our wait began. Court officials moved about. Spectators fidgeted in their seats. Counsel conferred with one another. There was some rustling of papers, but mostly we sat in silence.

The afternoon dragged on. Some people left. Once I caught

the eye of my detective friend, Lumsden, who raised his eyebrows and shrugged his shoulders non-committally. Then suddenly the court was called to order. The jury had reached a verdict. As they filed into their places I searched faces for some clue – a smile perhaps from one or other of them. Their faces were expressionless.

The judge seated himself on the dais.

"Have you reached a verdict?" he asked.

"Yes, my lord," said the foreman, standing. "We find the accused not guilty of manslaughter."

I saw Inspector Lumsden just once after that. I congratulated him on his perspicacity as a detective and on his decency as a man.

"You'll never get thanked, you know that," I concluded.

"That doesn't matter at all," he replied. "I uphold the law – and doing that can be a rough business. Horton deserved all he got. I've got no regrets in his case. But somehow I couldn't let the Briggs case rest. You'd be surprised at the medical books I've read these last few months! And finally I turned to you people."

"Just because we were their family doctors?"

"Well, that, of course – but I made a few inquiries first," he said with a grin. "Remember, doc – there was that reasonable doubt, and whether you're a copper or not, justice must not just *be done*. It must be *seen* to be done."

Chapter Four

It has been said that the shortest, most hazardous journey a human being ever undertakes is from the mother's pelvic brim to the vaginal opening.

That is a dramatic way of describing childbirth and there is

19

still a lot of truth to it, although modern technology has rendered childbirth a far safer process than it was thirty or forty years ago, when there were a few basic, well-established precepts. Those basics are still important despite the advances in technology. For instance, we judged the size of the baby relative to the measurements of the mother's pelvis. Was the birth likely to be an easy one? Was the baby too large, perhaps, to undertake this journey unassisted? Was a Caesarean section advisable? But our system of measuring was primitive and chancy, compared with the use of today's ultra sound where, without exposing the unborn baby to dangerous X-rays, the doctor can detect abnormalities in the fetus before it is born – and not just abnormalities in the baby's size or position in the uterus, but in various of its organs. This, and other methods of early diagnosis can detect possible complications long before they reach the stage of becoming dangerous to mother or child.

We know far more about our body chemistry than we did thirty or forty years ago and we know a great deal more about scientific baby care. Infants that would have had a very tenuous hold on life when I was a young doctor are often perfectly safe today in the hands of neonatologists (or specialists in the care of the newborn) in the specialized hospital wards to which such infants can be transfered at a moment's notice, even over long distances, by helicopter. Indeed, a "high risk pregnancy" can often be detected early enough that the mother can have her baby not just in her local hospital, but in a hospital equipped to deal with such cases.

The death rate amongst the newborn in technically advanced countries has been tremendously reduced over the years but at the turn of the century in Scotland, of every one thousand babies born, one hundred and thirty would not survive the first year of life. Despite modern technology, newborn babies can still face a hazardous time at birth and for a few days afterwards, but it is a far cry from my days as a young doctor, when babies were delivered at home, and we doctors had to rely often on our "clinical instincts" in making up our minds as to what we should do next in some unforeseen emergency.

Most babies are born without trouble. Having a baby is a natural event. It isn't an illness and shouldn't be treated as such,

20

although I remember when having a baby meant ten days in bed afterwards. I'm sure many a hardworking, overtired housewife welcomed the rest, but lying in bed does no good for the circulation, and many women ended up with clots in the veins of their legs.

When I first heard of the proposal that mothers should be encouraged to get out of bed almost immediately after giving birth, I was delighted. It was an innovation in treatment at the time, and I tried the new method on Mrs. Hodgkinson who had had severe thrombophlebitis following an earlier delivery. Mrs. Hodgkinson was enthusiastic too, and on the fifth day, to my surprise, I met her wheeling her twins up the street in their pram.

I stopped my car.

"Well!" I exclaimed, "I was just coming to visit you!"

"Don't bother," smiled my patient. "I never felt better. That business of having to lie in bed was sheer murder. But I'll tell you something, doctor, you're finished in this street. You'll never deliver another baby here," she went on, cheerfully. "The women all think you're an absolute brute getting me out of bed like that. Too bad," she grinned, "you have to pay the price for progress. But if my old man plays his tricks again, never you mind, I'll come back to you."

Mrs. Hodgkinson had had her twins at home. It was, luckily, an easy delivery. But the death rate in the delivery of twins is still about ten times that for single births. Nowadays twins wouldn't be delivered in a patient's home. They might not even be delivered in small hospitals with limited facilities. Doctors are often quite happy to transfer their twin deliveries to specialized units, for too much can go wrong with them and when things do go wrong, they tend to happen with catastrophic suddenness.

That's the trouble with delivering babies. For all our modern technology, nobody can say that this or that baby can be guaranteed to make its appearance without trouble. Every delivery has a potential for disaster and nobody can predict the outcome with certainty.

But even when all goes well, new parents sometimes don't know what to do about the firstborn when they've got it. As was the case with the Tompkins.

I had delivered Mrs. Tompkins a few days previously at their home. Mr. Tompkins was a schoolteacher. One who managed to make me feel I was back at school again. Indeed, I began to develop a distinct inferiority complex during the course of his wife's labor. Mr. Tompkins disapproved of my attempts at levity. He didn't like my seemingly casual approach to the business in hand. What he didn't know was that applied casualness was a technique I had used for years. His unsmiling eyes followed me everywhere and he had a quite unenviable gift for sarcasm in response to the most polite of questions.

Fortunately, it was an easy delivery. A few nights later, in the middle of the night, I was awakened by a thunderous knocking at our front door. I leapt out of bed and scrambled downstairs, clutching my dressing gown about me. As I raced for the door, I could hear the howls of an infant. It was heartrending and enough to rouse the neighborhood.

I opened the door. There stood Mr. Tompkins, attired in *his* pyjamas and dressing gown. Distraught, he thrust his newborn into my arms.

"For God's sake, doctor," he shouted. "*You* take it! It's been going on like that for an hour and I can't stop it."

I placed Master Tompkins over my shoulder and patted his bottom. There was a series of the most audibly satisfactory burps, considering the size of the bundle. There was immediate calm. My disparager of a few nights before stood there, his jaw agape.

"But – but what did you *do*?" he cried. "What did you *do*? It's been hell!"

"Mr. Tompkins," I said, "It's all done by the flick of the wrist. Here you are. Take him. Just explain matters to nurse tomorrow. *She'*ll make a professional out of you." And I retired to bed.

At the same time, mere "wind" in an infant can be no joke. We have had young parents phone us, distraught, because of it. We have heard the howling of babies in the background. It has gone on perhaps for hours before a mother has reached for the phone in desperation.

However, one chap who took all baby troubles in his stride, was one of our young associates in Hull, Raymond Thompson.

How I admired his calm competence, his refusal to be ruffled by the problems of the newborn. He was an example of detached, imperturbable efficiency, and I envied him for it.

I had the privilege of being the family doctor to one of Hull's specialists, Dr. Winston, a surgeon, and one morning I was called to his home. His little daughter, he told me, "had a bellyache" and would I "mind having a look". My "look" was brief. His kiddy had, I was sure, an acute appendicitis, and I joined my colleague in the kitchen, where he sat with his wife, neither of them saying much.

"John," I said, "I think your little one has an acute appendix. Would you care to have a look with me?" I knew my friend to be an expert surgeon. I trusted him totally.

"Gibson," he said. "Don't ask me to examine my own child. My judgment's no good where my own is concerned. You think it's an appendix, I'll give you the names of a couple of surgeons I have confidence in."

The doctor who treats himself has a fool for a patient, and my friend was a wise man.

It was around this time that I delivered Mrs. Kayrter of her first baby. Like all the rest, it was a home delivery. The midwife was in attendance, but I have never believed in arriving for the last ten minutes of action, delivering an obstetrical benediction to the newborn and leaving. I was in and out of that house with great frequency and before long it became obvious that this was not to be an average delivery.

Mrs. Kayrter's baby came face first. It is an uncommon presentation and one that is fraught with problems. In those days it was impossible to diagnose the condition prior to the mother going into labor, and I spent a most uncomfortable hour or two, but after something of a struggle, Miss Kayrter emerged, bawling, into a heartless world.

It would be fair to say that I developed a certain proprietory interest in the little creature after that, and when, a month or two later, just at the end of a long evening surgery one Friday, Mrs. Kayrter phoned the office and apologetically asked if I could call to see the baby, I was inclined to cooperate. Besides, the Kayrters' house was on Raymond's way home!

"Raymond," I said smoothly, "now you wouldn't mind doing this call, would you?"

"It's pretty late," commented my young friend, who had just been married and wanted to be with his wife. "Is it worth a house call?"

"Well I don't really know. But the Kayrters are nice folk. They never trouble us for trifles, do they? It'll only take you a minute or two to look at the babe," I pleaded.

"That's all right," said Raymond, who was easily placated. "But you know what I'm going to find, don't you?"

"No, what?"

"Anxious parents, that's what I'll find," he said, as he pulled on his coat, "and a kid with a bit of a temperature and a cold in the head."

The weekend passed pleasurably and when, on the Monday morning, I asked casually,

"What about the Kayrter kid, Raymond?" Dr. Thompson, who was busy going over his list of house calls, looked up with a grin and replied:

"Just what I expected – a kid with a bit of a temperature and a cold in the head," then went cheerfully on his morning rounds.

The months went by. The little incident of the Kayrters' baby was long forgotten, lost in the daily grind of work. Then baby Thompson arrived.

It was in the early hours of a nasty, drizzly, foggy east coast morning when the phone rang. It was our associate. Anxiously and apologetically, he said,

"I just hate to do this to you, Morris, but I'm worried about the baby. Would it be a lot of trouble . . . "

Off I went. Raymond met me at the door, wrapped in his dressing gown. Unsmilingly he said,

"Just go upstairs, Morris," adding, like every other young father, "I'll have a cup of tea ready when you come down."

Joyce, his wife, greeted me warmly, even smilingly, apologizing for disturbing my rest. Joyce, with her nursing training, seemed somewhat unperturbed as I examined their newborn.

Then I retired to the downstairs sitting room where my young friend had placed a tray containing a cup and saucer, teapot and biscuits for my comfort. He was hovering over it as I settled myself comfortably in his easy chair.

"Miserable night, Raymond," I remarked as he poured the tea. It was a cold night. The sitting-room fire had been out for hours. Raymond was a bit shivery, I thought, despite his warm dressing gown, while my heavy overcoat allowed me to ignore the cold night air.

"I am sorry, Morris, to get you out, but . . ."

"When were you thinking of taking your holidays? August, wasn't it? Nice month, August – especially up in Scotland. You'll enjoy it then . . . "

"Yes, Morris, but what . . . "

"This tea is lovely, Raymond," I went on as if he'd never spoken, "and those biscuits – simply scrumptious – I suppose Joyce made them hersel . . ."

"Never mind the bloody biscuits . . ." exclaimed my friend, "What about my kid – that's wha . . ."

"Oh, that," I said, in great surprise at his exasperation – "it's just what I expected – a kid with a bit of a temperature and a cold in the head."

The Indians have a saying that to know how a man feels about something, you have to walk in his moccasins!

Chapter Five

The wind from the North Sea was sweeping across the East Yorkshire plain, bringing with it a foretaste of winter.

It had been a busy week. I had seen many patients, but with the Sunday morning house calls completed, I had spent the afternoon working in our garden. There my digging, more for exercise' sake than from necessity, had given me pleasure. And I experienced one lasting little joy.

All summer two robins had shared the freedom of our garden and one had become steadily more brazen in his advances than the other, until he quite regularly perched at the foot of my wheelbarrow as I pushed it about. When I stopped, he would flutter to the ground and wait, hardly a foot away from my prodding spade, where he would pluck at the wriggling worms I exposed to his sharp little eyes. I used to whistle to him as I worked – soft, repetitive sibilances – and it seemed at times that we shared a kind of communion. If my worm production wasn't fast enough for him, he'd move away a foot or two, stand motionless, his head cocked to one side listening, then he'd pounce, adding another wriggler to the victim already in his beak.

My little garden friend was a British robin – a tiny creature compared with the North American robin, which, so they tell me, is scientifically classified as a thrush. That may be so, but they share one characteristic – cockiness.

Sometimes he seemed to listen to me, and I told Janet that one day he would be trusting and brave enough to hop onto my outstretched hand. Janet had often watched from the kitchen window, listening to the advances I made to my tiny companion and laughingly saying that he probably thought I was another very large robin.

But that Sunday afternoon my camera was dangling round my neck in readiness and I photographed my garden friend just as he hopped onto my trowel and clutched it with his tiny feet. It was a good beginning for the week.

When evening came, filled with the contentment that derives from physical work in the open air, I settled down before the open fire, the sheets of the Sunday newspaper cascading onto the floor around me. I pontificated on the state of the world or listed the films we ought to see, little heeding the gentle wind and the rain beating softly against the window.

And then the wind was no longer gentle, but a howling gale that rattled the door and whined around the house, and Janet said,

"Listen to that. What a dreadful night to be at sea."

I agreed, as I heard the wind lashing rain against the wall. And it was no surprise when Janet looked out and announced, "That's not rain any more. It's sleet, and in sheets."

Evening turned to night and the storm's fury grew. The wind whined eerily round the corners of the house, and the trees, lashed alternately by the force of the gale and the torrents of rain, swayed madly to and fro. I thought then of that afternoon, and hoped that my little bundle of feathers was safely hidden from the blast. But however secure he might be, he was a long way from the comfort of a blazing fire, the company of my little family, and the intellectual stimulus of *The Sunday Times* and *The Observer*.

Our daughter sat cross-legged on the floor, finishing her homework. Her notebooks and my newspapers made a casual melange on the carpet. All was quiet except for occasional brilliant political observations from me, and those were quickly quelled by Catriona's admonitory finger and the accompanying,

"Quiet, Dad, this homework is very important, you know."

The little one, her homework done, retired for the night. We listened to the late night news, then switched the radio off.

"All this trouble in the world, Janet," I remarked, "but thank goodness it's somewhere else nowadays."

Our partnership as a husband and wife medical team was a good one. We took pride in our work. We had prospered. Our garden was no longer a concrete backyard, but a beautiful lawn, bordered by a rose garden and a beech hedge. A little copse of blue spruce sheltered the house from the quiet road and, at the back, opening onto the crazy paving that led across the lawn to an old tree stump bordered by rockery plants, were the French windows. It was Janet's dream home come true, and that night we reveled in its warmth and comfort. Like Robbie Burns' character, Tam O'Shanter, in the security of his Ayrshire pub,

"The storm without might roar and rustle,
Tam didna' mind the storm a whistle."

And so to bed, basking sleepily in the warm companionship of my wife, drifting into glorious slumber, until the phone rang and all my senses were shaken alert.

27

"It's Missus 'oneywell 'ere, and Mister says you've to come at once. It's an emergency. Straightaway, 'e says."

I raised myself on my elbow and reached for the alarm clock. It was just after one in the morning! Outside, the trees bent with the force of the gale, and I heard a branch break off and crash to the ground. The rain and sleet rattled against the window, and it seemed only sensible to ask what the emergency was about.

"Never mind what's matter, you'll find out when you get here. Right now, 'e says." And before I could continue with the conversation the receiver at the other end was slammed into place.

I have always known the value of the doctor's visit. In North America it is often regarded as an old-fashioned and inefficient way of practising medicine. I don't agree. Many patients can be seen initially at home and even treated there. The benefits of house calls in terms of both treatment and knowledge can be considerable for doctor and patient alike.

But without adequate information, how does one assess the importance of a call? There was no point in my phoning back. The Honeywells, like most people in Hull then, didn't possess a telephone. The call had been made from a public phone booth a yard or two from their front door. Well I knew it! It had been used to summon me on a number of occasions in the year that the Honeywells had been "on our list".

Under the National Health Service, British patients join a doctor's list. They cannot go to doctors indiscriminately. The family doctor chosen will provide all primary care, with referrals to specialists in case of need. The doctors, in turn, receive a fixed sum of money per patient per year, whether they see that patient once, or a score of times. It is neither the best nor the worst system of payment in this world. For the patient, attendances at doctors' offices are "free". And the Honeywells had had more than their fair share. They had seen to that.

Swearing quietly, I got dressed. Tiptoeing downstairs lest Catriona should waken, I closed behind me the door to comfort, pulled my coat collar up and faced into the sleet. In the few steps to the garage door, my trouser legs were already soaked.

I backed my car onto the empty roadway. That automobile was not yet six months old. I had polished and handled it with all the loving care of a devoted owner. But through no fault of its own, it was to be unsteady transport that night. Within a hundred yards I had lost control of it. The road surface was deceptively icy. The car swerved, slid into the bank, hit a rock, rebounded onto the road, turned backwards and slid down the gentle incline until it came to a stop in the gutter. Fortunately, the road was deserted. On such a night only people with urgent business were abroad. My gloomy inspection of the damage confirmed my worst fears. The fender was bent and the body-work on the left side was dented and scratched from one end to the other. Gloomy, cold and wet, I clambered behind the wheel and slowly drove the mile or two to my destination.

If ever a couple belied their name it was the Honeywells. They were somewhere in their late sixties and had no family. They had been patients of ours for a year or so, and lived in one of those red-brick terraced houses that line so many English streets, just as British as the Union Jack. Their front door was flush with the pavement, a dark corridor leading past a small front room to the kitchen with narrow stairs up to the bedrooms. The rooms were cubbyholes but in many such houses they were also places of warmth and love. You couldn't have said that about the Honeywells'. Their house was comfortless. No pictures adorned the drab walls, although above the bed was the framed motif, "God Bless This Home". One felt it was more a demand than a supplication.

Mr. Honeywell was a fat man with a round, red countenance. On the face of it, he should have been jolly. He wasn't. His expression suggested perpetual, contained anger. His wife was as thin as he was fat, and equally pleasant.

When I got out of my car at their door, the rain had already run into my shoes. I didn't linger. I gave the knocker a sharp rattle and pushed the door open. A dressing gown over her spare frame, the lady of the house was waiting for me in the ill-lit corridor.

"You've taken your time, 'aven't yer?" she greeted me. "Oop stairs." She jabbed her thumb over her left shoulder in the direction of the stairs, then vanished into the kitchen, closing the door behind her with a slam, leaving me in the dark. I could see a shaft of light from under the door at the top of the landing, so lugging my medical bag I clambered up, knocked and entered. Mr. Honeywell was sitting up in bed. I noticed with concern that his normally ruddy complexion had turned a kind of dusky purple. His blood pressure had always been normal for a man of his age, and opening my emergency case, I took note of my patient, as a physician should. He wasn't coughing. His breathing was normal. He certainly wasn't collapsed. Mentally trying to make a spot diagnosis, I murmured, "a dreadful night, Mr. Honeywell," as I produced a thermometer and went to place it in his mouth.

My patient struck it aside.

"What the 'ell d'yer think yer trying to do," he roared. "There's nowt matter wi' me. It's 'im next door you've to go and see."

I was justifiably confused.

"But, Mr. Honeywell, it was *your* wife who phoned. Said it was *you*. She said this was an emergency."

"Aye, that's reet, an' you just go an' deal wi' it too."

"Mr. Honeywell, I don't understand."

"Well, if ye'd listen, ye'd understand. Can't yer hear?"

Through the wall, I could hear "The Mountains of Mourne" being scratched out on a fiddle. A very out-of-tune fiddle.

"I hear someone playing a fiddle, Mr. Honeywell. What's this got to do with any medical emergency?"

"It's 'im and that bloody vy-o-lin, that's the emergency! 'E's been playing it for hours and 'e won't stop. It's upsettin' my sleep, that's what it is, 'im and 'is bloody vy-o-lin."

"You mean to tell me, that this is what you have sent for? Because your sleep is being disturbed?" My question was as ice cold as my physical being.

"Not getting my sleep is part of it, but 'im playin' 'is vy-o-lin is upsetting my health and upsetting my nerves. I'm entitled to care for my 'ealth an' my nerves, so I am, so you go in next door and tell 'im to stop playin' 'is bloody fiddle. That's what you've to do. I've been bangin' on't wall for hours t' make 'im stop – an' 'e joost keeps at it."

The air around me was becoming sulphurous.

"On a dreadful night like this, I'm soaked through, my car is smashed, and I'm sent for because your neighbor insists on playing his fiddle?" My voice had risen to a roar. "Why didn't you get the police if he was creating a disturbance?"

"I've 'ad police, mister, and they say 'e isn't making a nuisance of 'isself, that's what they say. But I'm telling you, 'im an' 'is bloody vy-o-lin is upsetting my nerves, and I'm entitled to care for my nerves."

Speechless with rage, I closed my medical bag, and told Mr. Honeywell exactly what he could do about future medical care. I had almost reached the bedroom door, when the sufferer shouted at me:

"You just do as you're bid. You're a civil servant nowadays! You're paid to look after my 'ealth, so you just get yourself in there an' tell 'im to stop playing that bloody . . ." I had heard it the first time. On the verge of apoplexy, I delivered a harangue that left nothing to the imagination. I stormed downstairs and out, missed my footing on the curbside and stepped into the slushy, icy, foot-deep torrent that was roaring through the storm sewer.

As I slammed the car into gear, I suddenly thought of that robin. Somewhere he was tucked away as warm as a pie and without a care in the world!

In our travels Janet and I have met hundreds of doctors who, like ourselves, reluctantly left Britain to practise elsewhere. It was always, we found, a hard decision for anyone to make, and generally an irrevocable one, since with the advent of State medicine, doctors could no longer move at will from one practice to another.

It's an old story by now, and of no importance except as an explanation of the steps thousands of doctors took, especially in the fifties and sixties. Janet and I were a tiny part of the social revolution of "nationalized medicine" in Great Britain.

It has sometimes been said that a reactionary medical profession fought the scheme to the end, but in fact the majority of Scottish doctors and almost half of all English doctors voted in favor of a National Health Service. Janet and I supported this plan that would protect people from the ruinous effects of illness and the high costs of modern treatment, and in our experience, most doctors had active social consciences whatever their apprehensions about socialized medicine. But with state control came bureaucracy, which is not to be confused with intelligent administration or efficiency.

I was having supper one evening when a young specialist in surgery phoned me. As an elected official of the Medical Association it was my duty to support any complaints brought up by a colleague. He told me he traveled twice a week to a small hospital twenty miles or so from Hull, to remove children's tonsils.

"They've stopped my gasoline allowance," he said. "They've told me I've to travel by bus in future. It's all in the interests of economy," he said bitterly, "but I can get there in half an hour if I use my car. It takes an hour and a half with a bus wandering through every village in East Yorkshire. And then," he went on, "I have to walk some distance to the hospital. It's often raining, so I'm soaked and tired when I arrive. And I don't like the instruments provided. I prefer my own, so I carry my bag, and when I start operating my wrists are sore. On what they pay me I just can't afford to use my car to get there. It's all such a waste of time and efficiency," he finished.

I made a mistake. I'd had a bad day. My supper was getting cold, so facetiously I gave him a homily on the benefits of fresh air and exercise after days spent in the germ-laden atmosphere of a city hospital.

He'd never met me and didn't appreciate my remarks, although inwardly I too was seething with indignation over the stupidity of the situation.

"Sir," he said, "have you got any children?"

"One little girl."

"How would you like *her* to have throat surgery done by a man who is cold, wet, fed-up and has sore wrists?"

I made what amends I could, but it was no surprise to learn that he eventually went to Australia.

But rigid officialdom did not just affect us doctors. It sometimes humiliated our patients.

Roger and Betty Smith owned a little butcher shop. They were a devoted couple, content with little pleasures, and Janet and I felt deeply for them when Roger developed a cancer of

32

the liver. He knew what the future held for him and worked until he could work no longer, getting thinner, more jaundiced by the week, until finally disease conquered strength of will, and he took to his bed in their little home above the shop.

Betty fought on, but she had not trained as a butcher like her husband and customers began to drift away. One day, tearfully, with Roger sleeping in an adjoining room, she told me she was at the end of her tether.

"We've almost no money left," she whispered. "But Roger will never know. As long as I can keep going, we'll stay ahead."

"Mrs. Smith," I said, "surely you're collecting sick pay for your husband?"

"Oh no, doctor. You see, we're self-employed. We're not entitled to that."

"Look," I told Mrs. Smith, "since the change of government, that law has been changed. Self-employed people *are* now entitled to sick benefits – so you should apply."

She said she would, but two weeks later told me that her application had been denied, on the grounds that she had not applied within the prescribed time limit.

I offered to intercede, and phoned the official who had signed the letter. Had he really denied these people, I asked in my most conciliatory voice? And did he realize that Mr. Smith was dying, that his wife was at her wits' end? Yes, he did, he said, and there was nothing he could do about it.

"But surely," I said, "this is a special case? The Smiths didn't know . . ."

"Ignorance of the law," he snapped, using the phrase so beloved of jacks-in-office, "is no excuse."

"Mr. So and So," I purred, "my patient is dying. His wife is desperate. Now this lack of common humanity on your part seems to be the kind of thing that the London *Daily Express* would love to get its hands on. I'll phone them this afternoon." I put the phone down and waited. About fifteen minutes went by before it rang again. As I expected, it was my bureaucrat.

"Now don't do anything hasty, doctor," said my caller. "We'll . . ."

And he did. The Smiths got their money.

It was seven years later, with a sense of acute disenchantment and a feeling that I should turn to other, unencumbered professional pursuits, that I began to study law in my spare time. Janet, too, was discouraged and even suggested that we might buy a small hotel somewhere. But our Scottish stubbornness came to our rescue.

"I'll be damned if we'll be forced out," she said. "We've worked hard – we've achieved something – so why give it up?"

But seven years of frustration is a long time and in the spring of 1954, Janet, Catriona and I visited the United States and Eastern Canada. Undoubtedly it was a trial run.

From our base in Washington, D.C., we saw the real America, not the shallow, violent America of TV. We stayed in lovely old towns on the eastern seaboard, met decent, modest, kind people. Not once were we made to feel like foreigners.

I was offered work. In one lovely little village, people offered to support Janet and Catriona, find them a house, if I'd do the stipulated internship and practise there, even for a few years.

We had certainly warmed to the country, "But," I'd said, "it isn't home. I'm a Britisher and we're going back to Britain, to make the most of it, to settle down."

During the year that followed, I gradually realized that "making the most of it" was just not good enough.

Chapter
Six

Miss Gooderham was my first patient of the day. She was an attractive lass, and on a cheerless Monday morning, with low, leaden grey skies and a steady drizzle of rain falling softly against the windowpane, a pretty face was some compensation for the weather.

She was in her middle thirties, a blue-eyed blonde with a fetching figure and it was easy to answer her coy and wide-eyed smile.

"Good morning, Miss Gooderham, and what can I do for you today?"

Her reply, demurely pleasant, indicated no real challenge to my intellect and casually I listened.

"It's my hair, doctor. It just seems to be in very poor condition. I'd like you to prescribe something."

On the surface of it, this was going to be easy. Her hair, carefully coiffed, looked pretty good to me. On the other hand, people do worry about their hair. They sometimes get depressed when it falls out or turns grey. Men worry about becoming bald and grey-haired secretaries have been known to worry about holding their jobs in the face of competition from younger, prettier women.

But the condition of a person's hair can be a significant indicator of health. Many a doctor, seeing a patient's dry, thinning hair, has correctly diagnosed deficiency in output of the thyroid gland before the patient has said a word.

I decided to have a look at Miss Gooderham's scalp. Rising from my chair, I made my way to her side.

"Let's just have a look."

I lifted my hand towards her hair, but the lady, by gracefully moving her shoulders, deftly avoided my examining fingers.

"Oh! There's no need for any examination. All I really want is a prescription."

"But I have to know what I'm prescribing for!" I said. "So let me have a look at your scalp."

I could see I wasn't intended to disturb that coiffure, and patiently I assured her I'd be very careful.

"It's just a little dandruff," said the lady. She was right, too. There was no underlying rash. The scalp was healthy and so was her hair. Even the dandruff was minimal. Still, dandruff can be a nuisance and once established, can only be kept in check by regular shampooing. The only and final cure was suggested a century or so ago by an eminent French dermatologist – the guillotine!

I explained this to my patient with smiling good humor and reached for my prescription pad.

"I know just the thing . . ." I began, when I was charmingly interrupted.

"Don't bother to give me one of those Health Service concoctions," said the lady, smiling and rummaging in her handbag from which she produced a colored label, laying it on the desk for my inspection. "This is the stuff I want."

The face on the label stared back at me. It was a beautiful face topped by beautiful hair. At the bottom of the label were printed the words, "Super Miracle Hair Lotion".

Bemused, I looked across the desk at my patient. Her composed smile rested on my face.

"But, Miss Gooderham, this is a patent medicine! You can buy it at any druggist's for a few shillings! I can't prescribe this kind of stuff, *free* on the National Health Service."

She corrected me.

"You can't buy that stuff for a few shillings. If you'll notice, that's the *Super* Miracle Hair Lotion. It costs thirty-five shillings a bottle. *Regular* Miracle Hair Lotion costs three and sixpence."

"Miss Gooderham – it's a patent medicine. It may be very good, for all I know, but patent medicines are not on the list of drugs from which I can prescribe. Now," I went on, "I'll give you a prescription for a quite effective hair tonic."

Miss Gooderham's smile had vanished and so had her air of wide-eyed innocence. Not for the first time in my life I recalled that attractive women, when crossed, can become cold-eyed, thin-lipped, even menacing.

"Do I get this lotion? I'm entitled to it."

"Miss Gooderham, if the British public all felt they were entitled to the likes of Super Miracle Hair Lotion and Super Magic Stomach Balm, the Health Service would be bankrupt inside a year. I'm sorry."

She eyed me steadily. Those eyes, so alluring five minutes before, were as cold as ice.

"Didn't you hear what Mr. Bevan said on the radio two nights ago? He said that patients could get anything they needed from

36

the National Health Service if it would do them good. And," she added, "my neighbor said this is just the thing for me."

"Miss Gooderham," I interrupted her. "That's what some newspapers reported Mr. Bevan said. I don't think the Minister of Health was talking about Super Miracle Hair Lotion at thirty-five shillings per bottle. It's outrageously expensive, and furthermore," I went on, "your neighbor's pharmacological opinion doesn't interest me."

"Mr. Bevan . . ."

"Yes. Well, when Mr. Bevan puts it on the list, you shall have it. Meantime, I'm not going to charge this kind of thing to the taxpayers of this country."

Despite the fire in the grate, a noticeable chill had developed in the room. Miss Gooderham rose to her feet and made for the door. There she turned.

"Mr. Bevan said . . ." she began.

The waiting room door had been opened and closed so often that I knew I was in for a busy morning, and after that, I had a long list of house calls to be done. Some of those calls, I knew, were fairly urgent.

"I don't know what he said," I snapped. "What politicians say and what they mean are often two different things. I'm not giving you that stuff at the taxpayers' expense and that's an end to it!"

"No, it's not," said the lady, who departed, slamming the door as she went.

And back she came, a week later. She had patiently waited her turn. It was the middle of winter and the coughs and snuffles emanating from next door indicated the arrival of the seasonal flu. There was no cheerful greeting from either side as she made her way to the desk. The label for "Super Miracle Hair Lotion" was placed before me.

"I'll *have* a bottle of that."

"Sorry. I've checked the list of free drugs. It's not on it. You must buy it if you want it."

"Then I want to see a specialist."

"For dandruff? I'm not going to waste specialists' time for that. Do you know how overworked those men are? Besides," I added, "you've refused the treatment I offered."

"OK. I'll take your prescription."

I had won! Politely I gave her a prescription for a stimulant hair lotion, added advice on the use of shampoos, and ushered her to the door.

She returned within the week. Stonily she said:

"Your prescription was useless. Now I want to see a specialist!"

"Miss Gooderham," I said, "I'm a very busy man. We have a flu epidemic on our hands. You've not given any treatment a chance and furthermore, the National Health Service was not set up to cater to this kind of demand."

"I've looked into this," she replied. "Now, I've asked several times to see a specialist and you've refused to refer me to one. I've a good mind to complain."

Under the regulations of the N.H.S., family doctors were bound to refer their patients to specialists when necessary. Patients could not see specialists by self-referral unless, of course, they paid to see one privately. As far as her case was concerned, referral to a specialist was a waste of public funds and I said so.

"Very well. I'm going to complain direct to the Minister of Health and to the Executive Council. I have my rights. You'll hear more about this."

Having at this point told Miss Gooderham to find another doctor and realizing that this could take a month or two, I pondered my position. I was not unknown to "higher authority". I had no love for the growing intrusion of bureaucracy into our professional lives. I was, however, president of my branch of the British Medical Association and I could already see some of my political enemies licking their chops with anticipatory relish. A charge of failure to give adequate care might not stick, but the publicity could be damaging to me and by imputation, to all my colleagues, locally.

So I sent her to a skin specialist and gave her a letter explaining the case. Hurriedly scribbled letters were not for me. My letters had always been written with some pride, though for the past year or two, my reports had been getting pretty brief. And so, succinctly, I wrote about Miss Gooderham.

The specialist's reply was brevity itself. It was my own letter returned. Underneath my signature were written the words:

"For God's sake give her the stuff."

38

Miss Gooderham had brought me my colleague's reply. She stared at me in triumph as I opened the letter.

"Now, do I get it?"

"No, you don't. The specialist didn't prescribe it. He said I should. It's an outrageously expensive luxury and I do not believe it's allowable. But," I held my hand up at the sight of her enraged face. "I will seek the advice and opinion of the Health Service authorities. If they say you can have it, I won't argue."

And so, fairly, but forthright in my denunciation of such a waste of public money, I appealed to "the proper authorities".

The reply was written by some disembodied spirit who "felt" rather than thought. It took two typewritten pages to tell me what "it felt". It felt that:

"in section 109 of the regulations, paragraph 21, section 3, that . . ." and went on to let me know that "under paragraph so and so, subsection this and that, it *was felt* that . . ."

None of it made any sense, but the small print, invisible to most eyes, was easy for me to divine. It said:

"Back to you, doctor!"

I capitulated. I was working from morning till night. There were sick people to be cared for and babies to be delivered, usually in the early morning hours. Miss Gooderham retrieved her lotion as regularly as clockwork.

At the end of three months, my pay cheque arrived. In the envelope was a letter. There was nothing ambiguous about this one.

"In that you have, on a number of occasions," it began, "improperly and negligently prescribed Super Miracle Hair Lotion, which is not a medication approved by this authority . . ." It went on till it came to the point.

The cost of all the lotion obtained by Miss Gooderham had been arbitrarily deducted from my pay!

It was hard medicine for a Scot to swallow – surely I had treated the lady not just well, but most generously?

Much has been written about "doctor and patient." At one extreme their relationship has been enshrined as a mystical one, bound by the twin catalysts of personal privacy and professional conscience.

Like most young ex-service types I used to smile politely when older men talked that way. The services hadn't been too bothered about personal privacy, and yet most of us service doctors, I do believe, had kept a tolerably good relationship with servicemen. True, we were in a position of some authority.

At the other extreme the doctor-patient relationship has been described as a prosaic business contract and nothing more. I have never accepted that description either.

What there has to be between the doctor and his or her patient is mutual trust and respect. A relationship lacking those ingredients is likely to be fruitless, even antagonistic.

I was driving into Hull one dark, wet night. My Standard Vanguard was hardly a year old, and was an excellent car for city work, maneuverable and speedy when needed. My first new car after the war was a thing of beauty to look at – low-slung, fast – and a dream to drive on the open road. But it was not suitable for the stopping and starting every few hundred yards that is called for on a doctor's rounds.

Suddenly as I cruised along, I saw in my rear mirror the lights of a car coming up directly behind me at high speed. Before I could pull over out of its way, the car, which didn't stop, struck the Vanguard, sending it through a brick wall and into the canal. Fortunately, the car did not sink immediately. It had nosedived into the water, the police told me next day, and come to rest on a large oil drum tossed overboard by some passing ship. I made it to the bank and, soaking wet, walked towards a lighted police box, whose bemused occupant was staring along the dark and empty road.

"What the 'ell was that explosion?" he asked.

I explained the situation. The hit-and-run car was never found, but I was taken home. A police officer accompanied me to our front door which was opened by a pale-faced Janet. I hadn't realized that my face wasn't so much muddy, as bloody and muddy.

" 'Ere y'are missus," said my escort cheerfully. "It's a bloody miracle 'e's alive, so it is."

The car was a wreck but so essential a part of my equipment, that next morning I bought the cheapest replacement I could, and set off on my house calls. One of those was to the Bricknal home.

The Bricknals had been patients for years. I had delivered their two children and taken care of the family ailments. Our relationship had been friendly. I had prescribed for little Donald's bronchitis and was giving some last-minute instructions as I stood at the front door when Mrs. Bricknal looked over my shoulder, sniffed, and said,

"H'm. Another new car, eh? The one you had wasn't a year old. You doctors are doing just too well out of the Health Service – new cars whenever you feel like it. And *we* have to pay for it all."

I had a sore head and a lacerated scalp. I was not in a good mood.

"Mrs. Bricknal, do you remember Dr. Pullen who had our practice?"

"Yes. He was a good doctor."

I wasn't sure of the implication contained in her tone of voice, but I went on.

"They tell me he did his rounds in a chauffeur-driven limousine, an Armstrong-Siddeley, that he owned a Lea Francis sports car for his personal use?"

"That's right. He was very grand."

She said it with a certain pride and I have often wondered if the doctor who is "grand" and independent, isn't more impressive for some people than his less flamboyant colleague who merely tries to be competent and is paid from public funds.

Grimly I told Mrs. Bricknal that my Vanguard, through no fault of my own, lay at the bottom of the canal, that the "new car" she took exception to was the cheapest I could buy, and that my predecessor, without the taxpayers' or the State's beneficence, had done quite well for himself.

An apology was neither given nor requested, but because of such incidents, the yearning to be my own man once again grew.

Then one night, after a busy evening surgery, I was called to see little Elizabeth Dornton. She had a fever, said her mother, and would I mind "dropping in" on my way home, as if it were some kind of social occasion. Still, parents sometimes justifiably

41

worry about such things and cheerfully enough, I agreed to see the child. She had a mild respiratory infection. It was hardly any emergency, but I gave Mrs. Dornton a prescription, put my stethoscope in my bag and was heading for the door, when she said,

"Oh! Just a moment, doctor. Alfred's not feeling very well and he's not had a check-up for a year. We thought – seeing's you're here – that you might just give him a bit of a going over. He's in the bedroom waiting."

"What's the matter with him?"

"He's just a bit off-color. He's got his clothes off. He's waiting for you."

I climbed upstairs, satisfied myself that Mr. Dornton, aged forty, was not about to expire, suggested that he should come to the office for an examination and descended the stairs to be met by a Mrs. Dornton obviously displeased with the brevity of the consultation.

"I'd like you to have a look at this rash on my leg, doctor."

I looked, saw, scribbled out a prescription and made for the door.

"Oh no! You can't go yet. When we knew you were coming we sent for my parents. They're in the sitting room. All they want is their prescriptions renewed. It'd save them coming to the surgery. You're not required to examine them," said my patient, pertly.

Mr. Dornton had joined his spouse. They had been our patients since 1946. It was now 1955. And I was annoyed.

"Do you remember what would have happened before the Health Service in a case like tonight? I'd have charged you twelve shillings and sixpence – double the usual fee for an after-hours call, and you'd have paid it cheerfully as you always did. For my part, I would have carefully examined one sick child. But you'd have thought twice before sending for me, just because it would have cost you.

"Elizabeth isn't really very ill, and you know that. But you have demanded attention for five people – at this time on a Friday night. It won't cost you a red cent. It's an abuse of the Service and it's an insult to me. There's just nothing as cheap as something for nothing," I finished.

I looked at them. Then I asked them,

"Are you really happy with the service you get?"

"No, we're not," I was told. "For one thing you don't spend the time on us you used to."

"I agree," I replied, "that I no longer am able to spend time where it's needed. And *I'm* not satisfied either. And I intend to do something about it."

Medicine may be to some degree a science, but it is also a very human and personal art. Politicians in their attempts to impose doctrinaire or blanket policies tend to forget this, for blanket policies not only create problems but in some way or other they seem, whether in Canada or England, to destroy or damage the personal relationship that is so necessary for both patient and doctor.

In a reflective address, entitled "Government and Medicine", given to the Canadian Medical Association in 1961, Dr. Wilder Penfield, the eminent brain surgeon, said: – "some form of government assistance to people in regard to the costs of medical care is inevitable in these days of social consciousness."

He welcomed a National Health Insurance scheme for Canada but warned his audience of the pitfalls.

"It should make the patient very happy, the rich one as well as the poor, provided he does not lose thoughtful, friendly contact with his physician. No one wants to become a number on a card, whose medical case is reviewed by anyone who happens to be on duty. It should please the physician . . . if the scheme does not lose for him the ancient doctor-patient relationship – or the opportunity to move forward in the art of the practice of medicine."

For us, it all happened a long time ago and our decision was a personal one. I hoped that eventually there would be changes for the better, and despite all the vicissitudes of the Health Service, there have been such changes. British surgical and medical skills still rank among the best in the world and I have seen general practices that are models of humanity and competence. But at that time we did not see how, as family doctors, we were likely to "move forward" for years to come.

Chapter Seven

Our last few days on British soil were spent with friends in Scotland. All around us were reminders of the history of our native land. Our friends' home had been a fortress in medieval times and its stone walls were many feet thick. The battlements on the tower had been built with an eye to grim purpose, and if the main door was small and cramped for such a massive structure, it was not because of Scottish stinginess. The heavy door, once battered open, allowed entrance to only one man at a time and the narrow, spiral staircase had been constructed so that men retreating up it had the sword hand advantage over their pursuers.

Catriona slept in a huge, canopied four-poster bed that intrigued our excited little one almost as much as the stories of some of its previous occupants, but for Janet and myself the days were filled with thoughts and memories.

Soon it was time to leave. Our point of departure was to be Prestwick airport on the Ayrshire coast, and since we had been told that our flight was to be delayed for several hours, we decided to have a leisurely dinner in the airport restaurant. Although Prestwick had achieved the status of an international air terminal, it was still a small, almost intimate place, centered round the huts and hangars of the Second World War, when it had been a base for transatlantic military flights.

The restaurant was a popular venue for local people who enjoyed dining comfortably and well in the exotic company of world travelers. Air crews often ate there, the immaculate uniforms of the air-hostesses and pilots contrasting with the tweeds of casual diners and adding to the glamor of the surroundings. The restaurant building was airy, the windows wide, allowing the soft sun of an early Scottish evening to shine in. With its uniformed, attentive waiters, its thick carpeting on the floor and spotless linen on the tables, it was a welcoming place made warmer by the subdued buzz of genteel Scottish voices all around.

That dinner had a dreamlike quality about it for Janet and me.

Catriona, secure in our company, was all agog with excitement. We had been "processed" by the Canadian airlines people. There was no turning back, and I found it hard to believe that after all those months of worry, discussion, and apprehension, we would be quitting Britain within a few hours for the unknown challenges of practice in a Canadian prairie town.

Great Britain's financial problems of that time had led to very strict controls on money leaving the country. Like all emigrants, Janet and I were allowed to take only $400 apiece with us. My life insurance policy had been frozen and in the event of my death, Janet would have to return to Great Britain. It was not transferable to Canada. After our last few years of comfortable living, $800 seemed a small amount with which to begin life afresh.

As we sat quietly in the anteroom waiting to board our plane, its departure time now announced, we studied our fellow passengers. Transatlantic flights were still uncommon to the British at that time and our fellow travelers seemed to us a silent, reflective lot.

But Janet's attention fastened on a slightly built, elderly man who sat quietly by himself. She pointed him out to me.

"If I were a detective," she said, "I'd swear that man is a doctor."

"What makes you think so?"

"I don't know. Some kind of an instinct. Doctors often have a look about them."

But our conversation was cut short when a further delay was announced – one that would mean the airline putting us up overnight at the airport hotel.

Next morning at eleven o'clock, we finally boarded our plane, a Super Constellation, for the long flight west. Our good friends, anxious to be able to see us off, had stayed the night outside Prestwick and were now standing quietly on the tarmac waiting for us. Catriona was hugged and kissed and we grown-ups said goodbye.

It was a Scottish leave-taking, with more unspoken than spoken thoughts, quiet good wishes and subdued smiles as we climbed aboard, turned and waved before the plane doors were closed and we began our journey to Canada, a world away from Scotland's glens and castles.

It would be a long day: thirteen hours to Montreal then, as compared with the time taken by today's jets. For a very long time, we were over the Atlantic itself, the ocean's great crested rollers looking like waves on a children's yacht pond.

Janet and Catriona were seated behind me and after lunch, as I was reading that morning's *Glasgow Herald*, someone slipped into the seat beside me. He was a small, wiry, formally dressed gentleman in his early sixties, I guessed, the same elderly man Janet had remarked on as he sat by himself in the airport waiting room.

"Excuse me," he said, "I hope you don't mind, but I felt I'd like to speak to you. I was watching you while we waited at Prestwick. You aren't by any chance a doctor, are you?"

I was flabbergasted and amused.

"Yes, I am," I replied, "and furthermore my wife, who's also a doctor, had you spotted as one too!"

"She's quite right. And *I* spotted *you*. You're not going on any holiday either. You're emigrating, aren't you?"

"Yes."

"Where to?"

"Alberta. To a little town called Okotoks."

"My name is Johnstone," he said, as he shook hands with me and smiled at Janet. "Lloyd Johnstone, and I'm going to Toronto; and in a few weeks on to Alberta to visit my sister. She's getting on now, but she's still in practice – one of Alberta's pioneer doctors, I might say, Dr. Ruth Harvey of Olds. Olds is quite a bit north of Calgary. But tell me, why are you going to Okotoks?"

"It needs a doctor," I replied. How many times I had said that in the past few months! It had been the only brief yet adequate answer to many a question.

"Then there's no better reason for going there," replied my new friend with great conviction. "I know of Okotoks," he went on. It's a very small place, but presumably the town council must be pretty sure the area can support a doctor. There's no hospital there, is there?"

"I understand there's a hospital in the town of High River, about fifteen miles south."

"Yes. You'll be required to undertake hospital work, you know," continued my friend, thoughtfully. "Have you kept up with it at all?"

"I've done no hospital work since 1948," I replied, "and not because I wanted it that way," I added.

"Yes," said Dr. Johnstone. "I'm sure of that. That may present you with some difficulty when it comes to joining a hospital staff, you know. But that's a bridge to be crossed when you come to it."

"Dr. Johnstone, I can't quite place your accent," I asked. "You don't sound quite like an Englishman or a Canadian."

"Perhaps I'm a bit of both," he replied, smiling. "I'm a Canadian. My background is partly Scottish, but I went over to Britain during the Great War, served with a British regiment and after the war I stayed in England, trained as an eye surgeon and for many years I've had rooms in Harley Street."

He didn't add that he'd been highly decorated for gallantry or that he spent months of each year in the Far East as a medical missionary, doing eye surgery. He and his wife, a tiny, indomitable Scotswoman, devoted much of their life in "retirement" to curing blindness in the poor of faraway places.

He seemed to read my thoughts.

"I suppose your funds are frozen?" he asked.

"Yes, and that worries me," I confided to him.

"Don't let it. Have you a letter of introduction from a bank manager?"

"Yes, I have."

"Then see the banker in Okotoks or Calgary. Canada is a very young, flexible country, the West even more so than the East. You'll be all right, don't worry," and having said that he walked back to his seat.

At long last, after another delay of several hours at Montreal, we landed at Toronto, the first lap of our five-thousand-mile journey over. Dr. Johnstone came to say goodbye and introduce us to his cousins, before he was cheerfully whisked away.

"Courage!" was his parting injunction, as we shook hands.

It was two o'clock in the morning and steamy hot. Bedraggled travelers sat on overcrowded, shabby, brown leather settees and stared into oblivion or shifted uneasily in their sleep, crooking their heads in their arms as they tried, quite hopelessly, to work themselves into more comfortable positions. Around us was the raucous noise and bustle of the airport, with taxis constantly coming and going, doors slamming, people greeting one another, announcers calling out flight times and the steady roar of engines, as plane after plane took off and lumbered up into the darkness.

It was an abrupt, almost an alarming change from the quiet gentility, the calm of Prestwick airport. But it was different, exciting, even at that early morning hour.

"God!" I thought, "but they're a rough-looking lot!"

There was a tall, lanky Westerner, stetson tilted carelessly to the back of his head, wearing a fringed buckskin jacket over blue jeans that almost concealed his western riding boots. He was being stared at by his fellow countrymen, I noticed, but then! – he was the width of a continent from home, a fact that a Britisher "just out" might find difficult to comprehend.

Husky men wearing multi-colored shirts and carrying lumber jackets stood beside their gunny sacks, the ubiquitous blue jeans tucked into heavy, calf-high boots. They were transient workers, engineers perhaps, on their way to some distant project in the wilderness. Shirt-sleeved businessmen, their collars and ties loosened at the neck in forlorn attempts to keep cool, folded jackets into some semblance of pillows and tried to sleep. Tired-looking women tried to keep children in order. And surrounding us, that motionless, all-pervading, damp heat.

The country, of course, is so vast that the only practical way to travel any great distance is by plane, and even in the early fifties, people traveled by air in a casual way that was foreign to most Europeans.

"Here," I thought, "is immense vigor. Rough it may be, but it has a vitality that hits you right between the eyes."

Chapter Eight

At Toronto we learned that our plane for Edmonton, the capital of Alberta, still two thousand miles away, had gone. We were assured we would be put aboard the first flight west.

Some time passed before a flight attendant told us a plane would be leaving shortly, that we could board at once. We gathered our suitcases, glad to leave the steamy heat of the air terminal for the walk across the tarmac to the waiting plane, but there was no relief in the open air. It was as hot and humid as a well-kept greenhouse.

We were tired and yet excited as we boarded our North Star, one of the work horses of Trans-Canada Airlines – now Air Canada. It was a heavy, propeller-driven affair – slow, by today's standards but, so I've been told by pilots, immensely reliable, with its four Rolls Royce engines.

Safety belts fastened, we waited. Almost continuously planes kept wheeling into line, the roar of their engines rising to crescendos as they lumbered up into the night sky, their lights rotating, the blue flames of the exhausts showing up the outlines of wings in the darkness. Then we were off, rising and banking over the myriad lights of the city beneath us, as we turned and headed west. A cheerful flight attendant brought us blankets and pillows.

"But," she said apologetically, "this is really an unscheduled flight. Since the transatlantic flight was so late, it was decided to put you aboard this plane. I'm sorry to tell you we don't have prepared meals aboard, but we'll find you something to eat. And there's no water in the lavatory taps. It's going to be a milk run. We refuel at Winnipeg, then it's straight through to Edmonton."

We were too tired to care. We dozed restlessly until touching down at Winnipeg. There were perhaps half a dozen other passengers aboard and I was glad to stretch my legs while Janet and Catriona slept. The air was still hot, but while there was almost a metallic smell to it, it was crisp and dry, no longer oppressively humid, and I welcomed the change.

From Winnipeg we flew over the prairies. They stretched endlessly to the west, the earth brown, flat, and divided into great squares by the road allowances running geometrically north and south every mile. And if the land had been divided geometrically, it had been plowed geometrically too. These great square fields bore no resemblance to the lush green farms of England. The plains as far as the eye could see were almost treeless, with snow still lying in some of the gulleys where the warmth of the sun had not penetrated.

The rivers were grey gashes on the face of the earth, wandering raggedly on their way, the same a hundred miles to the west as they had looked a hundred miles behind us. Here and there, thousands of feet below, farmhouses stood stark and alone. Even at that height it was obvious that they were of basic design. Some of the buildings were surrounded by trees, obviously planted as shelter from the winds; other buildings stood alone, isolated on the bald prairie, at the mercy of snow, wind and sun. Many of them, I would later learn, were the huts built by the first settlers: frugal homes devoid of any of the comforts to which we had become accustomed.

Janet and I said little to one another. We were both absorbed in our private thoughts. And even our little one was quiet as she sat beside her mother, silently surveying the panorama beneath us. We were entering a world different to anything we had known before – vast, bare, harsh, empty.

But when we touched down at Edmonton there were houses around us, and smiling people, and the warm, beautiful early summer sun of Alberta. The air, still chill, was like dry wine – crisp, refreshing.

We were directed to the airport hotel. What we needed was sleep, and I asked for a room. We must have looked an incongruous trio when I think back. Since we could bring little money with us we had seen to it that at least we were dressed in the height of fashion. Janet looked a dream in her London suit and coat. Catriona was as smart as a little ticket, and as for me, I was another dream – a bleary-eyed one. I had bought a natty gent's double-breasted suit, fashionably striped in contrasting colors, all of which was topped by a light grey homburg hat, the likes of which I later realized hadn't been seen in Edmonton since Queen Victoria's Jubilee. The dazzling effect of my tailoring was a little spoiled for the desk clerk as he surveyed our entrance. I hadn't shaved recently; my sleep had been fitful, my mental state wasn't exactly placid and I probably looked as if I had been on the bottle for a week.

"And what can I do for you folks?"

"We need a room."

"Right now?" He glanced at his wristwatch. "We won't have a vacant room for hours. I'll see what I can do later in the morning."

"Can we have some food?"

"Now that's something we can fix up. Excuse me asking, but you people look all in. Where have you come from?"

I explained the situation, how our transatlantic flight had missed the connecting flight and how we had traveled across Canada on a "milk run". Our questioner was galvanized into sudden action.

"You just come with me," he said. "Breakfast is coming up. Come and sit by the window here. And so you're emigrants from the old country. Great! You'll love Canada. You're staying in Edmonton or going somewhere else?"

It hadn't occurred to him to ask what kind of a job I might be going to and I simply told him we were going to Okotoks, twenty-five miles south of Calgary.

"I know Okotoks," he said, "and I sure know Calgary. I used to live there. And I know the old country too. I was four years over there, mostly with the Calgary Highlanders. You've got friends in Okotoks, of course, that you're starting out with?"

"No, we're going there to start up."

"Start up what?"

So I told him. He had already ordered breakfast for us, given Janet a cup of coffee and our little one a huge glass of orange juice. He nodded thoughtfully as he listened.

"I think you could do better for yourselves than Okotoks. It's not a town by British standards – more like a little village. No paved roads. The last time I was there it didn't have any running water – just shallow wells and outside privies. Mind you, that's some years ago. It may have changed. But I'd look around a bit if I were you."

51

The deliciously fried eggs and hashed potatoes the waitress had placed before me suddenly became indigestible as I listened to him, and he sensed my dismay.

"Look," he said smilingly, "you three are going to love Canada. And we need all the Britishers we can get. Now eat that food. I'm just coming off duty. I'm going to find you a nice, inexpensive hotel downtown and I'm going to take you there. I'll be back."

Within minutes he returned.

"I've booked you in at the Corona Hotel," he said. "I'm just going to bring my car to the door."

Our flight bags vanished. I called for the bill.

"Oh," said the waitress, "that's been taken care of."

Adamantly she refused my money. The desk clerk, she said, would be very upset if I insisted. And he was waiting at the door for us.

The drive downtown took minutes. That airport is still there; nowadays it is used for local flights only. Edmonton International Airport, suitable for a growing metropolis, lies twenty miles to the south in the quiet countryside.

At the door of the hotel, our friend unloaded the luggage, helped me carry it into the lobby, and turned to leave.

"Please let me pay you," I pleaded.

"There's no way I'll let you pay," he grinned. "Many a meal I was given in the old country. This has made my day, so don't try to spoil it. Good luck, Catriona," he smiled down at our little one, extending his hand in the western Canadian way, while Catriona shyly took it. He shook hands with Janet and me, and with a wave, he was gone.

I registered at the hotel desk.

"We won't have a room for an hour or two," I was told, when a voice behind me said,

"You must be the people from the airport." It was the manager, and he added, "You all look exhausted. Come with me."

We trudged upstairs.

"Take a seat," said our guide, as he stood at a door and knocked. Then, in an aside to us, "These guys won't mind being disturbed."

There were seven or eight men inside, holding a conference of some sort.

"Gentlemen," said the manager, "I've got three people here from England. Their plane connections went wrong, and they're dead beat. Could I move you out of here and put three beds in instead? Go and have a coffee and I'll find another spot for you, I promise."

I waited for protests, but none were forthcoming. The men trooped out. They were about my own age, and as they stood around, one or two of them introduced themselves, shook hands, and began to talk.

"How's London these days?"

"Piccadilly the same as ever?"

"How's old Glasgow town?"

"Has it ever stopped raining at Greenock? I used to go in there with convoys. I never knew a dry day at Greenock the whole of the war."

Beds were being wheeled into the room as we watched. There was a buzz of conversation, questions, reassurances that we "had done the right thing" in emigrating. In the end we had all shaken hands, a western custom that before long became second nature to me.

Too tired even to thank our host for his kind efforts on our behalf, we tumbled into bed and slept.

Chapter Nine

It was late afternoon when we wakened. The sun's rays were streaming into the room. We bathed. I shaved and felt twenty years younger for that little ritual. We changed our clothes and eagerly set out to explore Jasper Avenue, Edmonton's main street. That first impression of Alberta – of broad streets and sunshine – remains to this day.

Janet, not surprisingly, had lost her lipstick somewhere en route. Why women feel unprotected and exposed without a lipstick I will never know, but we went into a chemist's shop to buy one. The druggist, as we quickly learned to call him, was a friendly fellow, and within a few minutes he had discovered why we were in Alberta.

"Okotoks!" he said, then, "Doctor, perhaps you should think twice about Okotoks. I'd like to help, and I bet I could find you a job with one of the clinics here inside twenty-four hours."

We thanked him but told him our minds were made up. We were going to Okotoks.

As we were leaving the shop, he hurried after us. "Just a moment," he said. "It might not work out the way you think. Here's my card and phone number. If you change your mind, phone me."

Gratefully, and thoughtfully, I accepted his offer. Next morning we presented ourselves to the registrar of the College of Physicians and Surgeons of Alberta. It was an important interview, for although our qualifications and required references had been forwarded by mail and tentatively accepted, the registrar had the legal authority and duty to interview us and satisfy himself that the public was protected from improperly qualified people. Certain standards of training had to be attained, and even after all our traveling, the official retained the power of veto, and he told us so. It was, at first, a frosty interview. He was distant but courteous, watchful and inquiring. We presented him with the required certificates of good character from the registrar of the British Medical Council, his opposite number in London. He accepted Janet's and read it quickly, scanned mine and murmured,

"Well, I see you have a record of fifteen years of undetected crime," but he was smiling as he said it, told us our official licences to practise medicine would follow us to Okotoks, and politely ushered us from his office. We were "in".

Our next visit was to the Edmonton office of the Immigration Authority. We introduced ourselves to the officer on duty, who listened poker-faced to our statement that we were eager to

54

proceed to our ultimate destination by the first available train. We were thinking in British terms of trains to here, there and everywhere every hour or two. We had a lot to learn.

"There is only one available train," he explained. "It leaves in an hour or two. The next one leaves tomorrow. And it only goes as far as Calgary."

"But of course there will be a connection from Calgary to Okotoks?" I asked.

"I don't know if you'd call it a connection. A train goes through there sometime tomorrow. There might be a bus. I wouldn't know."

The immigration officer had been looking us over as he spoke. He took in Janet's chic London suit, coat and hat and Catriona's demure schoolgirl clothes, but it seemed to be my gent's double-breasted blue suit and light grey homburg hat that caught his eye the most.

"Look," he said suddenly, "I'm on duty here today. Here's the file on you people, and I want you to know I made no arrangements about you going to Okotoks. Maybe somebody else did; but I'm going to give you a piece of advice – don't go."

"But we've agreed to go to Okotoks," I exclaimed. "We've come nearly five thousand miles to go there. We were told it needed a doctor."

"Oh!" said the official, "I've no doubt it could do with a doctor – but can it support one? It's had four or five doctors in and out of the place in the last five years. They all stayed a few months. People have got used to going to High River, the nearest town, or into Calgary. You just won't make a living, and that's the truth."

Speechless, Janet and I looked at one another. The official pursed his lips, tapped on the desk with his pencil, looked at me and said deliberately,

"Can I say something else? Can I put it straight to you? You won't make it in Okotoks, doctor. You're not the type."

I looked at him.

"What do you mean by that?"

"It's written all over you," replied the immigration officer. "You're a city doctor. It's in your file. Just look at the way you dress! You're all city people. You'll be lost in a town like Okotoks, all of you. Let me look around up here. I'll get you a job in a day or two."

I was staggered, but it was Janet who took up the challenge.

"We came to Canada to go to a town that needs a doctor. We were told Okotoks needs a doctor, and that is where we're going."

The official nodded, unsmiling. "Don't say I didn't warn you," he said.

I had one final word.

"You are the second or third person since yesterday who's tried to put us against Okotoks. What's wrong with the place?"

"Nothing that I know of," replied the official. "It's just that it's small – only six hundred and eighty people. It's the kind of place that doctors – mostly young, single men – move in and out of because they can't make a living there. That's all. It's not much of a town. Have you ever seen a prairie town?"

"No."

"Well, Okotoks is no better or worse than most of them. It's not like a pretty English village, believe me," he added. "But if you've made up your minds, I'm not going to stop you. Just remember – I'm here if you need me. I'm going to make inquiries, and I'll be able to relocate you pretty fast. I suppose you'll go to Calgary by train. Just let me warn you. You're going to see the backside of every town between here and Calgary – wooden shacks, outside privies – the lot. Don't be put off by the rail trip. It's not as bad as all that. But if Okotoks doesn't work out, phone me."

Our interview was over. Stunned, I ushered my wife and daughter into the sunshine – that warm, bright sunshine that saved our bacon that summer.

Catriona made my day. She had listened to it all, quietly and so maturely, for a little girl. Taking my hand, she said,

"Daddy, you *are* the type," while Janet with equal emphasis said,

"We're going to catch that train."

Calgary lies one hundred and eighty miles south of Edmonton. It was a long train ride. The immigration officer had been right.

We saw the drab side of the few intervening towns where grey, unpainted wooden houses, many of them shacks, lined the railway tracks beside the stations. Many of the towns – villages, in British terms – had no paved roads. As the train clattered over the level crossings, we could see that the roads had gravel surfaces, with the dust rising in clouds behind every passing truck and car.

Grain elevators, identical wooden towers painted in bright colors, stood in rows beside the tracks. The stations, like the towns, had a strange similarity to one another. They had none of the sense of order and permanence one associates with British towns.

They were settlements, collections of buildings hurriedly erected for purposes of convenience and shelter. Little thought had been given to design in terms of either architecture or organization. I've since seen the same kinds of towns in the country in Australia – dusty streets lined by wooden houses.

And that makes the point. We did not yet understand that we had come to a new country. Eastern Canada had long been settled. It was older, and two thousand miles away. In the East there were comfortable, modern homes. But only seventy years before, those little towns we were passing through had been collections of shacks, with perhaps a tepee or two nearby. They were dependent on the railway. If, in its development, it passed them by, they would die away. Other settlements would be built beside the rail tracks. We were seeing the surviving settlements of those early times.

Settlers, seventy years before, were just beginning to push into the prairies and foothills to undertake the back-breaking and often heartbreaking work of homesteading. Their neighbors were nomadic Indians – Blackfoot, Cree, Blood, and others – many of whom had never seen a wheel.

The great, unfenced prairie stretched for eight hundred miles from Calgary to Winnipeg. Seventy years before, Alberta was not yet a province. It was the untamed land, still the Northwest Territories, dependent for law and order on the "red coat policemen" as one old-timer called the Mounted Police.

We were still to discover these things. It was difficult to take them all in.

Three days before, we had dined in the comfort of a Scottish hotel. Now, as the train rattled along, we looked at the rolling countryside and the vast blue sky of Western Canada and wondered what lay ahead. Even in 1955 the West was just beginning to open up. We would see that happen.

But we would see the old West too, for we had come at the end of an era.

Chapter
Ten

When we reached Calgary it was mid-afternoon. It was the first Saturday in June, 1955. I had spent my thirty-ninth birthday over the Atlantic. We had left behind us one of those beautiful English springs, with daffodils in bloom, the spring colors bursting all around us, and were now about to greet our first prairie spring.

Certainly the sun was beautifully warm, the skies cloudless – but where were the spring colors? The scattered trees we had seen on our train journey from Edmonton stood out hard and severe against the sky, with not a bud or a leaf in sight. The grass was brown, lank and drab.

"As far as I'm concerned," remarked my better half, "we might as well be on Mars."

We had to learn that spring in the West is but a name. Summer seems to explode at the end of winter. The grass one day is brown and dry and suddenly one morning it is green.

But my immediate concern was transportation to Okotoks.

"Speak to the travelers' aide," said the train conductor when I asked him about ways of getting there. "There isn't any train till tomorrow. I don't think there are any buses either. But the aide may be able to help you."

I doubt if they have "travelers' aides" any more. They used to be an institution, in Western Canada at least. Generally they were older people, and many seemed to be volunteer workers. They were conspicuous in every railway station, sitting in their tiny, distinctively marked booths, ready with helpful advice about lodgings and transportation. Many a lonely traveler has had cause to bless them.

Our "travelers' aide lady" as Catriona called her, was a little wisp of a thing, elderly but as bright as a bee. Primly she assessed our needs, pursing her lips and adjusting her spectacles in her concentration. Having heard of our plans, she emerged from her little box of a booth, directed me to put our luggage beside her chair, closed and locked the gate and led us to the main door of the station.

When I think of it, by British standards, Calgary's railway station was a little box of a thing too. The passenger area was completely enclosed, which I thought a bit odd, and the whole place was tiny for a city of Calgary's size. What we had not realized was that this station dealt with perhaps half a dozen passenger trains a day – and as for being closed in, we still had to experience a prairie winter. British railway platforms are often dreary, miserably cold places on which to wait for trains, but at least travelers don't stand in danger of losing their toes or noses from frostbite.

We trooped after our "travelers' aide lady". Stopping at the main door she commanded us, "Go straight down that road," pointing across the street. "You will come to the Carolina Restaurant. It's very nice. Go and have a cup of tea and a cookie. Give me half an hour, then come back."

Having said that, she turned and with that quick little stride of hers, returned to her booth. "I'm going to do some phoning," she called to us as she turned away.

We were the best part of five thousand miles from home. My apprehension about the whole situation was steadily mounting, but that little woman, with her concern, her precise, matter-of-fact attitude to our problem of the moment, was a godsend. We had that cup of tea and the cookie. Refreshed, we returned to her office.

She had tried unsuccessfully to find people who might be driving back to Okotoks and who could give us a lift. We could stay overnight in Calgary, she said. She would find us reasonably priced accommodation.

"Let's take a taxi," said Janet, "and get on with it."

Already some of our money had gone, but a taxi would be worth the expense. After all, we had arranged to go to Okotoks. We were expected. It was only twenty-five miles away, so why spend another night away from our destination? We gathered our luggage and found a cab.

"Where to?" asked the driver, disinterestedly.

"Okotoks."

There was sudden animation as the cabbie looked round to see who or what was in the back of his taxi.

"*Nobody*," he said, "ever takes a cab to Okotoks!"

However, we soon convinced him that we really meant what we said, and he started off. He was not a very communicative taxi driver, but in answer to our query, he told us Calgary's population was about 160,000.

The road was under construction. We bumped and lurched along from one pothole to the next.

"What road is this?" I asked.

"The MacLeod Trail." Not a word was wasted.

"Why is it called the MacLeod Trail?"

"After some guy in the RCMP."

It was only later we would learn that the road followed a trail that is part of Alberta's history. The "guy in the RCMP" was Lt.-Col. James MacLeod of the North West Mounted Police, the legendary force that became the Royal Canadian Mounted Police.

In 1875 a force of 275 officers and men of the North West Mounted Police gathered in Winnipeg, then a settlement of a few thousand people. Their orders were to cross the uninhabited prairies to establish detachments, to enforce the law, to parley with the warlike plains Indians.

James MacLeod was an officer in that force, commanded by Colonel George French. The "North West Mounted", trained and uniformed in the manner of British cavalry, completed an epic journey in good order, despite the loss of men and horses en route. MacLeod distinguished himself as a leader and led his detachment to establish Fort MacLeod in what would later become southern Alberta.

What scenes there must have been in meetings between Indian warriors, restlessly moving about on their ponies, rifles and lances at the ready, and MacLeod at the head of his ordered ranks of mounted policemen.

But MacLeod's honesty and respect in his dealings with the native people became legendary. He never broke a promise. In 1877, just a little more than eighty years before our bumpy ride along the road that bears his name, MacLeod met with Chief Crowfoot of the Blackfoot confederacy. It could have been peace or war.

Statesmanship on both sides carried the day. Canada was spared the Indian wars that plagued the United States.

At that time, there was a lonely police outpost eighty miles to the north of Fort MacLeod, close to the junction of the Bow and Elbow rivers. MacLeod named it Fort Calgary which, in the Scots Gaelic, means "place of clear running water". Today it is a major Canadian metropolis.

That "guy in the RCMP" had accomplished quite a bit in a few years.

By now we were leaving the outskirts of the city. There were fields on either side of us. The houses were thinning out. We trundled over the railway crossing at Turner siding, where a wandering bear would be shot later that very week. We were into open country, approaching the hamlet of Midnapore.

"Midnapore," I repeated. "That's the name of a city in India!"

"Yeah," replied the taxi driver, "I believe you're right. Some guy that had lived in India gave it its name. There's nothing there. A few grain elevators and some houses near the railway track. But if you get a bad night with snow blowing, and you're on your way back to Okotoks from Calgary, you'll be mighty glad to see the lights of Midnapore. At thirty-five below, you just don't run out of gas on this road."

It was a warning, and a timely one, of things to come.

"Now there isn't anything between here and de Winton," he went on. "The new road isn't planned to go through de Winton, but it's another place to remember. I'll show you the turnoff."

We drove in silence for a few miles. We were entering the

foothills now, the road climbing enough to let us see on our left the great panorama of the prairie just beginning – flat, almost treeless and stretching for eight hundred miles to the east. On our right, the first gentle foothills unfolded one upon another. There were a few scattered farmhouses breaking the natural contours of the land, but I could see why the letter sent to us in Hull had described the country surrounding Okotoks as "sparsely populated". Still, it was a lovely day. There was hardly a cloud in the sky, and I marveled at the immensity of this great empty land.

"Last lap," said the driver, "just beginning."

The road curved to the right. I could see it unfold in front of us, dead straight, up one hill and down another, then up and down again, out of sight. That road, it seemed, went from one hill to the next and on into infinity.

"How far away *is* Okotoks?" I wondered.

"Look to your right!" commanded the cab driver.

We had rounded the bend and come out of the shelter of a hill. Before us stretched a sight that will live with me forever. Forty or fifty miles away to the west and stretching north and south for perhaps a hundred miles that we could see, stood the Rockies.

The snow-capped peaks stood out, stark and magnificent, against the blue sky. The serried ridges were snow covered, but on the lower levels the rock face, discernible even at that distance as great gullies and cliffs, was colored in delicate shades of purple, blue and grey.

"Daddy! Look! The Rockies!" exclaimed our little one, excitedly.

Janet, with a laugh, began quietly to sing,

"It's springtime in the Rockies,

The Rockies far away . . . " then interrupted herself with, "but I never ever dreamed I'd see them!"

Now I focused my attention on that road again. Up one hill and down another, that graveled road seemed to stretch into eternity. How far away *was* Okotoks?

Suddenly, on the brow of a hill, we were looking down into a valley. There was a river, shining in the sun, threading its

way between trees. There were colored roofs, and houses between the trees, and a street or two.   \

The taxi drew up at the crossroads.

"Okotoks!" said the driver. "You're home."

Home!

Depositing us on the sidewalk, the taxi turned in the middle
of the main street and in a swirl of dust was gone, heading back
to Calgary. As we stood there at the corner, our flight bags on
the roadway beside us, I looked at my little family and not for
the first time in the last few days, wondered if I was quite mad.

What in the name of heaven had driven me to leave a prosperous medical practice, and drag my wife and daughter five
thousand miles away to this little town about which I knew
nothing?

It wasn't the time to ponder the matter. I squinted down the
sun-drenched main street, taking in the graveled road, the few
false-fronted buildings that lined it and behind us, the old colonial-
style Willingdon Hotel. It all looked as if Buffalo Bill might ride
down the street at any moment.

"Come on, people," I said as cheerfully as I could. "Let's find
a room and then I'll go and see the Chamber of Commerce.
They'll have the whole thing straightened out in a jiffy."

We tramped into the hotel lobby. It was lined with dark wood
paneling; the floors were bare and echoed to our feet. Four or
five men in blue jeans and stetsons were sitting in a corner
playing cards. Their gunny sacks were piled in a heap beside
them. A suitcase was doing duty as their card table.

They stopped their game long enough to inspect us silently
before returning their attention to the cards. The wall on one
side of the lobby was graced by a very large old print. It showed
the *Empress of Canada* sailing majestically on a calm Atlantic,
and how I wished we were on her – going east! The dining
room, however, looked spacious and inviting, its spotlessly white
tablecloths a contrast to the dark paneling.

Joe Miller, the proprietor, was the first person I met in that
little town. As I told him who we were, I slowly began to realize
that as far as he was concerned, we might be visitors from outer
space.

"I'm delighted to hear that we've a new doctor – in fact, two

63

doctors – ma'am," with a slight bow to Janet, "but to be honest, this is the first I've heard of it."

"Ah!" I said, "I'll need your help in contacting the Chamber of Commerce. They're the people who arranged it all with the Canadian Immigration Service."

"Chamber of Commerce?" repeated Mr. Miller. "I've never heard of any Chamber of Commerce – at least not in this town. Chamber of Commerce?" he repeated in his puzzlement. "Doctor – let's get Mrs. Gibson and your daughter into their room and then I think you should cross the road and talk to the druggist. If there's a Chamber of Commerce in this town, he's the man who'll know about it."

We were shown upstairs to our suite. It consisted of adjoining bedrooms, of which the larger overlooked the main street. The wooden floors were uncarpeted, the brass bedsteads looked as if they had been there since the hotel was built at the turn of the century and so did the print on the wall, a large over-flowered English garden with cottage.

Little was being said by now, and feverishly I set out to interview the pharmacist.

"Where," I asked him, "do I find the Chamber of Commerce?"

"There isn't one," he said.

"There must be!" I exclaimed, and once again I explained myself.

The druggist seemed preoccupied.

"But," I insisted, in desperation, "the Okotoks Chamber of Commerce wrote to the Canadian Immigration people, who wrote to us, telling us the town needed a doctor. My God! We've come five thousand miles to practise here! And now nobody seems to know anything about us – or this Chamber of Commerce!"

"I'll phone around," said Mr. Berry, the druggist. "Will you be in your hotel room?"

I walked back to the hotel. Mr. Miller met me in the lobby.

He was a big man, a veteran of the Royal North West Mounted Police. They had a splendid reputation for rock-like imperturbability, and if Joe Miller was typical of them, this reputation had been well earned.

"Did you get it straightened out, doctor?"

"No."

"My wife tells me," he said, "that there was some talk a while back of forming a Chamber of Commerce in the town, but nothing seemed to come of it. I'll phone around."

"Phoning around," as I later learned, was one Canadian way of getting rapid action.

I rejoined my family. Silently Catriona and Janet were unpacking our bags. I sat in a chair and watched them. There was little else I could do. I don't know how long I sat there without speaking, except for perfunctory remarks about items of clothing. I wasn't in a conversational mood.

Probably an hour passed – a very long hour. Then there was a knock at the door. I opened it. Three gentlemen stood outside; one was Mr. Berry, still wearing his white druggist's jacket. One was a tall gentleman dressed in western shirt and frontier pants. The third was a man of about my own height, dressed in a business suit.

"I found the Chamber of Commerce," said Mr. Berry.

They filed into our room and introduced themselves. The tall man was Jack Meston, a real estate agent. Frank Pow, the smaller of the two, introduced himself as the manager of the local branch of the Royal Bank of Canada.

Having procured chairs from adjoining rooms, they sat down. There was sudden silence.

"Let me tell you," I began, "how pleased we are to see you people. We'd begun to think there'd been some terrible mistake."

It was Jack Meston who replied.

"To be honest, doctor, I think there has been. We're not expecting anybody."

My jaw must have dropped – visibly, for Mr. Meston hurriedly said, "Oh! It's all right. We're happy to see you – but we've had no word from anybody about you people coming here. We've made no preparations. We're completely taken by surprise. We've no place to put you, and," he added, "we had a quick get-together before we came up – there isn't a house for rent in the whole town."

Janet and I looked at one another, aghast. Catriona, a quiet observer, sat silent.

65

"And there isn't anyplace that'd be suitable for a doctor's office," Mr. Meston continued. "There isn't a single office space with running water."

"But you had actually applied to the authorities for a doctor to come here?" I asked, bewildered.

"Oh yes. We did. But we never got any reply. If we had, we'd have had something set up. But at the moment I hardly know what to say!"

Frank Pow, silent till now, joined in.

"We'll get things straightened out somehow," he assured us, to which Jack Meston replied,

"You bet. We'll start working on it right away."

"The town needs a doctor," said Mr. Pow, "and now we've got not one, but two, we'll just have to get moving. We've got to do something to help you people."

"That's right. We'll do something," said Mr. Meston. "Could you stay in the hotel for a week or so while we look around?"

"We've had Okotoks on our minds for months," said Janet. "It's a strange feeling to realize there's nothing here at all for us."

"There is, though," said Frank Pow. "There's a town that needs a doctor. I know it's a small place, but I can tell you that in wintertime it's very difficult for folks around here to get medical help. In fact, there have been one or two tragedies that might have been avoided if we'd had a doctor in town. And the same applies to the farmers in the district."

"It's seldom that doctors get here from Calgary or even from High River – that's our nearest town, fifteen miles to the south. Even fifteen miles is a long way at thirty below, and when a blizzard blocks the road it's impossible. We sure need what you two people have to offer."

"Can we make a living? – that's the point," I said. "We've been told we can't."

Jack Meston nodded. "I can see why some people would tell you that. But we've not just jumped at this. We've talked to a lot of people. We couldn't get hold of the mayor, but he agrees with us, and he'd be here with us if he could."

"We believe," said Mr. Pow, "that a doctor could make a go of it in Okotoks. There's a couple of thousand people in the area. After all, Dr. Ardiel practised here for many years. He died a few years ago, and since then we've had several doctors, in and out."

"Doesn't that speak for itself?"

"I don't think so. The community needs a doctor. I believe it would go out of its way to support the right one. Won't you give us a few days while we put our heads together?"

It was late afternoon when our visitors left. When they did go, I wandered round that hotel room, looking at Catriona and Janet, hoping that neither of them had noticed my mounting anxiety.

Suddenly Catriona cried, "Daddy! Daddy! Come and look! A *real* cowboy is riding up the street!"

We crowded at the window. There, below us on the graveled road, a horseman in blue jeans, western shirt and stetson, booted and spurred, his lariat neatly coiled on the saddle, was passing by. His dark complexion and raven black hair made him look very much part of the scene. I later made his acquaintance. He was called Pepper Cheyenne.

So even if we didn't see Buffalo Bill ride down the Okotoks main street that day, we saw the next best thing.

But eventually it was dark and we retired for the night, with Janet and Catriona sharing the front room while I occupied the room next door. I could not sleep. After hours of tossing and tumbling I slipped into their room to look at them. Janet was fast asleep but Catriona was awake. I saw those violet blue eyes follow my restless movements. It was almost dawn.

She beckoned to me, finger over her lips and very quietly I knelt beside her.

"Now Daddy," she whispered, "whatever you did, you did it for the best. And Mummy and I are *right with you.*"

Having said that, she put her arms round my neck, kissed me, and said, "Now please go to bed and sleep, like a good boy, for it's going to be *all right!*"

Chapter
Eleven

On Sunday morning we set out to explore the town.

The old part of Okotoks lies in the valley of the Sheep River. To the north of the river, a long ridge shelters the valley and the town from the worst of the sub-arctic winds of winter. The Willingdon Hotel still stands at the main crossroads, at the foot of the "Okotoks hill", a notoriously difficult place for vehicles in wintertime. The main business street runs east and west. That morning, for no particular reason, we walked towards the east end of town.

It was a mistake. There wasn't a soul in sight. The town appeared to be deserted. The wooden, false-fronted shops, stuccoed or painted in various colors, were closed. The Royal Bank, a two-storeyed brick building, dominated the north side of the street. On the south side there were several buildings, among them a hardware store and a butcher's shop, but there were vacant spaces in between, with crumbling basements and weeds growing through the cracks in the cement. We later learned that years ago a fire had swept along the street, destroying businesses which had never been rebuilt.

A couple of hundred yards took us beyond the business section and soon we were passing wooden shacks, old, grey from weathering and lack of paint, some of them leaning just a little to one side or another, dilapidated, yet lived in. It was not a cheerful stroll. What grass there was around us looked dead. It was old and yellowed. There were a few scrubby trees here and there, stark and bare, their scrawny branches silhouetted against the yellow brown of the bare hillside. An abandoned wooden theater, leaning just a little forlornly, was a reminder of Okotoks' past grandeur, when – so Mr. Miller had told us – the town had boasted several hotels and livery stables and rivaled Calgary in size.

Janet and Catriona were bravely smiling, but I swallowed hard as I remembered our home and garden at West Ella, with the daffodils, the soft lawn and that lovely copse of evergreens just beside the house. But *I* had burned our bridges behind us. There was no going back.

Suddenly a car drew up beside us.

"Strangers in town?" asked the driver. "Can I give you a lift?"

"No, thank you. We're just walking."

"Staying at the hotel?"

"Yes. For a few days."

"I'm Bob Mitchell," said the driver, a pleasant-looking fellow of about my own age. "My wife and I own the Okotoks Variety Store – and I'm not doing anything special for an hour or so. I'll be happy to show you around, if you've the time to spare."

His friendliness was infectious, and very shortly we had left the town behind us and were heading into the countryside.

We had driven from a seemingly deserted town to an equally empty countryside. We had not passed one person on foot, nor seen a single individual working in a field. There were no pretty hedges bordering fields, just barbed wire fences. There were scattered farmhouses, some of them standing stark and lonely in the middle of fields, others surrounded by belts of trees, as bare as the houses they were meant to shelter. But when Bob Mitchell stopped at the top of a hill and we stood by the roadside and looked around us, it was the immensity of the landscape, as well as its barren loneliness that overwhelmed us. The quietness was profound.

The undulating foothills to the west, like great land waves, one upon another, rolled against the first range of the Rockies, standing hard and grey against the skyline forty miles away. To the east, as far as the eye could see, was the prairie, treeless, flat, brown, lonely. It would be like that for eight hundred miles. Above us was that immense dome of blue that is the western sky.

I was used to the lonely, misty moors of Scotland, and to Yorkshire's dales, but this was different. The Yorkshire dales can be bleak, yet beautiful in their own way, just as the windswept moors of my homeland can draw a man back to them, but this was like no other land I had ever seen. And yet, I thought, there is a beauty too; but it is a harsh, lonely and perhaps a cruel beauty.

I said that to Bob Mitchell. He took no offence at my frankness. He nodded. He was looking up the river, sparkling in the sunshine. A few hundred yards away a couple of fishermen were placidly casting. Bob was watching them.

"Yeah. I agree with you. It sure isn't your cozy old country view. But it's beautiful. And it'll get better. We've had a long winter. The trouble is, it's all getting spoiled."

"Spoiled?"

"Yup. Too many people. Just look at those guys cluttering up the river."

For the first time in days I allowed myself a smile, but hastily smothered it when I realized that Mr. Mitchell was not being altogether flippant!

"And now," he said, "we're going back to have a cup of tea at my place."

While Mabel Mitchell produced tea and muffins, there was a sudden flurry of talk. Bob knew his England and, like so many Canadians, loved it. He had served there and in Italy as an infantryman. He had uncles and aunts in London, and he wanted to know the latest news from the country he had fought for.

A month later, with our friendship cemented, I told him how much we had appreciated his kindness that Sunday morning. Chance meetings like that one, I said, can have important results.

"Chance?" grinned Bob. "There was nothing chancy about it. I knew damn well who you were. I happened to see you pass our window, and I said to Mabel, "if these three see those shacks along the road there, and think that's what the rest of Okotoks is like, we'll never see them again. They'll just keep walking till they get to Regina. I'm going after them."

That afternoon we wandered along the hillside overlooking the town. We took care to go west! We could see trees, quite large ones, by the riverbank and along the valley. And there were trees in well-tended gardens surrounding cheerfully painted, comfortable-looking bungalows. It was dry and the sun was warm. As the three of us strolled along hand in hand, we noticed that we had company; a pretty, dark-haired, dark-eyed little girl of about eight years of age was wandering along the hillside, a few yards from us.

When she came close by, Janet exclaimed,

"What beautiful wild flowers you've got there. I've never seen flowers like those before! What are they called?"

The kiddy held out her posy of flowers for Janet's inspection.

"They're called shooting stars," she replied, "and they come out just about now – before it gets really hot. But you've got to look for them in the long grass!"

"As," said my wife, "perhaps we always have to look for the beauty that's hidden all around us."

"Yes," said our little acquaintance, sagely. "P'raps that's true. But please, don't you come from the old country?"

"Yes."

"My mummy comes from the old country," announced this little lady, "and she'd love to meet you."

Suddenly, impulsively, she ran up to "my two women", took them by the hands and cried, "Please come with me to meet my mummy," and began to tug and pull them down the hill. In the end she persuaded us to follow her to one of those tiny bungalows in the street below us, telling us en route that her name was Wendy Palmer and that her mummy was a school-teacher.

Pat Palmer, a tall, pretty, graceful woman, showed no surprise when we arrived on her doorstep. In a soft Irish voice she told us not only that we were welcome, but that we must stay for dinner.

Janet and I still remember that dinner – the luscious ham and mashed potatoes, the welcome we received, and the talk that accompanied that meal. Pat Palmer had not had an easy time since coming to Canada.

"But it's the people," she told us. "I'd never have managed without them. I've never known warmth and kindness like it. You'll find the same. Canada's a wonderful country."

The troubles Pat had overcome made my problems look miniscule. And she emphasized, like other people we had spoken to, that in wintertime especially, there was a real fear of accidents or acute illness, for sometimes the town could be isolated by blizzards. We were really needed, she said.

71

That night, before I fell sleep, I wondered if, after all, there was a future for us in that little foothills town.

What a difference a day can make.

Chapter Twelve

We stayed in the Willingdon Hotel for a week – a strange, dream-like week without work or the kind of responsibilities we were used to. News, however, spreads rapidly in such small communities, and we had visitors who shyly introduced themselves: a rancher who lived ten miles out of town, and whose wife had recently had a heart attack; and a couple whose diabetic child had become comatose the previous winter and had nearly died. If we would stay, they said, they would speak to neighboring farmers and ask them to support the new Okotoks doctors.

In that week, Mr. Pow arranged for me to have a loan of $2,000, confidently calling it an investment on his part, and Jack Meston found a house for us to rent. As he said, it wasn't much of a house, but it was a start. There were two tiny bedrooms, a small living room and a surprisingly large kitchen, dominated by a huge old-fashioned wood stove, "converted to gas". When Janet saw it, she told me, all she could think of was the attractive, modern Aga cooker she had left in Hull. It wasn't an encouraging sight, but then, neither was the news from England that our "settlers' effects" which should have followed us by ship, were lying in a dockside warehouse, and would probably stay there for another three months. There had been a dockworkers' strike.

We moved into our new home. Mr. Miller refused to take a penny in payment for our stay at the hotel.

"You've been my guests," he declared. "This town needs a resident doctor and this is my contribution to the community effort to get one."

Our brass plate bearing the words "Drs. Wm. and J.B. Gibson," had adorned the door of our surgery in Hull. Sentiment ordained that we bring it with us for our "office" in Canada, but since it was with those "settlers' effects", a piece of wooden board, neatly painted, and fixed to the front gate of our little garden, would do quite well.

We were in business. The trouble was that we couldn't find an empty office. For three months, our kitchen did duty as one. Nor was it at any time overcrowded, for people were still uncertain that we would stay in Okotoks, and why, they said, should they desert satisfactory doctors in High River or Calgary for this unknown couple? It was understandable.

So to begin with, we saw emergencies only. Our first patient had accidentally hacked his shin with an axe – a nasty injury that required more care than any surgical skill. Our second was assisted into our kitchen by a fellow ranch hand. The injury in this case was a little more complicated and quite a change from the "office cases" we were accustomed to seeing in Hull. This horseman had been riding through brush, looking for cattle that had wandered away from the main herd. One of the cows bolted and he had ridden after it, spurring his horse into a canter. Unfortunately he had neglected to wear the leather chaps that give protection to riders doing such work in rough country, and as he turned his horse, a branch of bush broke off, tore through his blue jeans and pierced his right upper leg.

He was pale-faced, shocked and in pain as he limped into the kitchen and lowered himself onto a chair. There was a trickle of blood down his leg and the least movement of his thigh increased his pain. Part of the branch was embedded in the wound, and at first sight the penetration seemed to be deep.

It was the kind of injury that in England we would have sent to the casualty department of the nearest hospital, but this was to be our first lesson in the ways of country doctors in Western Canada. They were expected to be capable of dealing with such emergencies on the spot. The two men looked at us expectantly.

Janet and I held a little conference in the sitting room, devised a plan of action and returned to our kitchen-office. First an injection of demerol, a morphine derivative, to ease the pain and lessen the shock. Then began the process of removing the piece of wood from our patient's thigh. Gently we probed the wound with our surgical instruments, carefully boiled on the kitchen stove for the operation. Fortunately when the branch pierced his leg it had traveled in an upwards direction so that the wood had not penetrated deeply enough to involve such vital structures as nerves or major blood vessels. Still, it was a nasty wound; the branch had broken off, leaving a couple of inches of wood protruding from the opening, which luckily was quite wide and allowed us to explore the damage. Carefully, we eased out the remainder of the wood, to the accompaniment of a few groans.

Then we set about the work of cutting away shreds of skin and fat that lay messily around the wound opening.

Such injuries always have an element of danger in them. They can become infected, however careful the cleansing process has been, and there is a risk of tetanus developing in people who have received no protective inoculations. However, when we had finished our work, we felt reasonably sure that all contingencies had been anticipated, and the patient, grateful for our efforts, departed.

If he was grateful, so were we – for the healing powers of Nature. His injury improved quickly and without any of the complications that might have arisen.

In a week, the countryside was transformed. Those scrawny trees we had seen were now in leaf, and they had a delicacy about them I'd not appreciated before. The river rushed through the valley, a thing of untamed beauty, swirling in torrents against banks that days before had looked dry and crumbling and now were green and lush.

We had settled down emotionally. We would consider our stay in Okotoks as a holiday. If we had to, we would get in touch with the Immigration people and move.

It was our first Saturday in our new home. I was just about to suggest a walk along the hillside when there was a knock at the kitchen door. Our visitor was a large man. He was wearing heavy boots and was dressed in khaki shirt and trousers, this ensemble topped by a stockman's hat. His trousers were held in place over a capacious abdomen by a leather belt with, as extra support, a pair of "policeman's suspenders", or braces. Set in an unsmiling face were two of the flintiest blue eyes I have ever had inspect me. And they were doing that as I said,

"Can I help you?"

He didn't answer immediately. He continued to look at me, then over my shoulder at Janet who was busying herself in the kitchen.

"You are the new doctor?"

"Yes."

"The name's Sparrow," he declared. "Jack Sparrow. I live here. May I come in?"

"Certainly, Mr. Sparrow."

Mr. Sparrow doffed his stetson and nodded politely to Janet.

"Ma'am," he said, before turning to me and shaking hands. Mr. Sparrow was a big man, not so much in height, though he must have been getting on for six feet, but in girth. I immediately sensed that even now – probably in his early sixties – here was the kind of man not to "tangle with", as the locals would say. There was an impression of strength, power, formidability, that made me wary.

But not wary enough. His hand simply engulfed mine and squeezed till my knuckles cracked. Squeezing back didn't help. I was about to whimper for release when he let go. He appeared to be quite unaware of my agony and I had no intention of mentioning it.

"Mr. Sparrow," I said, wondering if my hand would ever return to normal, "what can I do for you?"

"Remove a tooth," he replied without preamble.

Now, I had never removed a tooth. Dentists removed teeth, and I said so. Mr. Sparrow acknowledged that normally such was the case, but today, he reminded me, was Saturday. Okotoks did not possess a dentist, Calgary was twenty-five miles away, a dentist would be difficult to find at the weekend, and he was a busy man.

"I can prescribe some pain-killing tablets for the weekend, Mr. Sparrow, and then you could see a dentist on Monday."

"I've been in pain for two days, doctor. I'm not going to wait till Monday. *You* pull it out."

75

I was beginning to get a little edgy.

"Mr. Sparrow," I repeated, "it's a job for a dentist. I am not a dentist."

"I'm aware of that – but you are a qualified physician and surgeon?"

"Certainly," I replied with dignity.

"Duly licensed to practise Medicine and Surgery in the Province of Alberta?"

"Indeed yes." I could sense it was time to make a concession: "I am not a surgeon in the specialist sense of the word."

That was one of those British understatements you hear about. I hadn't been in an operating room for years.

"I understand – but you are qualified to carry out minor surgical procedures. Is that not correct?"

"Yes, of course."

This fellow, I thought, talks like a barrister-at-law.

"And you would agree that pulling a tooth is a minor surgical procedure?"

"Er-er, yes."

"And I presume you brought a selection of suitable surgical instruments with you?"

At this point, Janet tactfully left the kitchen for the sitting room, there to follow the rest of the consultation with growing interest and alarm.

I'd been caught out once or twice when giving medical evidence in court, made to feel highly uncomfortable by counsel for one side or the other, and Mr. Sparrow was causing me considerable discomfort now.

"So," he said, "what are we waiting for? Pull the goddam thing out!"

He sat in one of our plastic and steel kitchen chairs, leaned back, opened his mouth, stuck a large finger in and said,

"Ig's ish yun heagh," adding, when he removed his finger, "It's loose."

To my horrified eyes that molar looked about the size of the Rock of Gibraltar, and every bit as unstable. What in heaven's name was I to do? At the same time, I had gradually suspected that I was being tried out. Was I man or mouse? Mr. Sparrow,

76

at a later date, and in a more expansive frame of mind, was to confirm my suspicions.

And then I had a stroke of veritable genius.

"Mr. Sparrow," I said, smiling with Satanic triumph, "this is a very large, septic molar. I could not possibly think of extracting it without an anesthetic. We do not as yet have the equipment to administer an anesthetic. You will simply have to wait until you get to a dentist."

"I'd thought of that," replied Mr. Sparrow, nodding his head reflectively. "I'd thought of that. So I've brought my own anesthetic."

As if by magic, he produced from his hip pocket a large flask of whisky, opened it, gulped down an alarmingly large amount, corked the flask, put it on the kitchen table, leaned back, smiled for the first time and said,

"And now, I'm fully anesthetized. Just get it out before the anesthetic wears off, doctor."

Despair, desperation and determination drove me. I produced my instruments. I pushed, pulled, twisted, gouged and wrenched. I had to stop several times while more anesthetic was administered. My hands became clammy from my exertions and my terror. Loose? That tooth seemed to be embedded in cement. I will say this for my patient – he was a stoic, even encouraging me when my determination began to fade.

And then, suddenly, what had once been a gum rendered up the prize. The tooth, black, the roots as gnarled as the branches of some ancient oak tree, lay in my surgical basin. Exhausted, I sat down.

Mr. Sparrow was exploring his mouth with his tongue. He nodded at me.

"You got the bugger!"

Speechless, I nodded back.

My patient reached for the whisky. The flask was half way to his mouth when he put it down, looking at me, I thought, in a most peculiar way. Was he going to faint now – at this point, I wondered despairingly?

Suddenly Mr. Sparrow leaned forward, thrust the flask into my hand and said, "Here, you take it. By the look on your face, you need the anesthetic a great deal more than I do!"

Chapter Thirteen

Two months had passed since our arrival in Okotoks, and patients were beginning to arrive regularly at our kitchen door, perhaps four or five each afternoon. Despite all Jack Meston's efforts, there was no sign of any place we could use as an office.

Something had to be done, we agreed – but what? The problem was solved by a summons to visit Glen House at his home. Mr. House, a town councillor, was a tall, slim, elderly Texan, a handsome, rather stern man, grey-haired, aquiline of feature, steady-eyed, dignified, quiet.

It was said that as a young man, he and his brothers had left their lands in Texas and, driving their cattle before them across the great plains of the American West, they had eventually arrived in Canada's prairies, three thousand miles from their home.

He never mentioned his boyhood years to me, though many a tale he told me of his later experiences in the foothills.

"Ah!" he'd say, slowly shaking his head and looking over my shoulder into the shadow of the years, "but you'd have loved the West of my youth, doctor."

Mr. House was one of Okotoks' colorful characters. Louis Fleuret, the town secretary, was another. Louis, a cultured, dapper Parisian and a university graduate, had apparently served with the French Foreign Legion, and charming and friendly though he was, Louis was equally uncommunicative about his youth.

Mr. House greeted me with the usual handshake and bade me be seated. I had not met him before that day and as I sat in his comfortable armchair, I studied him. He, in turn, was watching me.

"I hear you're working from your kitchen, doctor?"

"That's right, Mr. House. I'll be glad when we can find a suitable office."

"I'm sure you will, and that's why I sent for you. There's an old one-roomed school sitting out in a field near the town. I could buy it for $500. It's very old – still got desks sitting on the floor. It'd do for a start – better than nothing."

"Mr. House," I replied, smiling, "there wouldn't be much point in seeing patients in the middle of a field!"

It was my host's turn to smile.

"We'll move it, doctor. I guess you don't move houses in Yorkshire. But we do it here all the time. If you're agreeable, I'll lend you that $500, interest free, and we'll arrange a town bee. We'll put the building on wooden skids and haul it right into town. We'll have a cement foundation ready, hoist it onto it, and there's your office ready-made."

He sat back and waited for my reply. It was a bit puzzling to me.

"Where would you put it?" I asked, "and how could you haul a big building like that several miles into town. And how would you hoist it on to foundations without cracking the thing apart?"

"You'll just have to watch the operation," replied Mr. House, smiling. "In the meantime, I should tell you that the town council is anxious to see you settled. Then you and your wife will stay, you see! So this offer is my contribution to keeping you both. Now, we've given a lot of thought to this, and the town council would be willing to give you and your wife a building lot just east of the hotel, if you'll accept the suggestion of moving the Skye Glen schoolhouse onto it."

"The Skye Glen schoolhouse!" I repeated. "The name alone should seal the bargain. My wife's father was born on the Isle of Skye."

A week later, we watched as three farmers drove into town on their tractors, hauling behind them the Skye Glen schoolhouse. It had been pushed and pulled onto long thick logs or skids, and was moving slowly down the street. A dozen men had donated their services for the occasion. Power and telephone lines were elevated so that the building might safely pass beneath them, and with the minimum of fuss and trouble it was winched into position on the prepared foundation. Mr. House stood beside us as the building was slowly but steadily eased on to the concrete.

It wasn't much to look at. It was old, grey, weatherbeaten and worn, windowless at the front that faced the street, but it was part of the history of Okotoks, and if its looks were bleak, there was nothing but warmth around us as spectators shook

79

our hands and wished us well. We had made a gesture. That day was a turning point. We had shown that we meant to stay.

The Skye Glen schoolhouse would continue to serve the community. It had to be divided into waiting and consulting rooms and extra windows had to be installed, but painted in warm colors inside, and modernized outside with its facing of log planking, it would see its share of human drama, joy and tragedy, for years to come.

Before too long, the practice began to grow. It was still a leisurely business, but it gave us time to collect our thoughts.

Sometimes, if old folk needed to have laboratory tests done at the hospital in High River, I'd take them with me and bring them back – or neighbors would. There was no public transport to High River.

"What was Okotoks like when you first came here?" I asked Mr. Minue as I drove him to the hospital one morning. "You're one of the area's oldest settlers, aren't you?"

"Yes, I'm certainly one of the oldest living settlers," replied my patient, a man well up in his eighties. "And it's strange that you should ask because I was just thinking last night that I believe I built your office. It was a one-roomed schoolhouse, you know, and they taught everything and everybody in that one room, from toddlers to young people. It was all done by one young lady teacher just fresh out of training. Those teachers were hardly any older than some of their students, and some of them were terribly lonely, coming from Ontario sometimes. They just didn't know what they were coming to."

We were crossing the Sheep River bridge, a steel girder affair, functional and devoid of any claim to beauty, but to our left lay the Okotoks public park and the river. The park was unspoiled woodland, with a small picnic ground, and paths wandering through the bush. The area was dominated by tall cottonwood trees, their thick trunks and stout branches showing through the clusters of leaves, gold and red in the autumn sun.

Mr. Minue was alone with his memories and I did not disturb him as he looked at the trees.

"They're lovely in their fall colors, aren't they?" he said in passing. It was a statement more than a question and silently I nodded my acquiescence. "Yes," he went on, "I'm sure I built your office. I had no education myself worth speaking of, but I could use my hands. Settlers were beginning to come in – men with families, not just young adventurers, and we needed a school, so I set to work and built one. Strange that it should be your office now, after all those years lying forgotten in a field! But you noticed those cottonwoods back there? When I came out here, that's where the Indians kept their dead. They laid them out on platforms up in the trees, all held together by thongs of buckskin."

"I suppose we all have our customs, Mr. Minue. I hadn't heard of that one."

"Oh! It's all long forgotten, I suppose," he replied, "but it was more than a custom. It made good sense. They couldn't have dug graves in winter with the ground as hard as concrete, and up there, they were safe from coyotes."

"What was Okotoks like?"

"It was just a collection of shacks – shacks and a few tepees. There were as many Indians as whites."

"Did the Indians resent you being there?"

"No, I truly don't think they did," he replied. "We whites kept mostly to ourselves and so did they, but we all got on well enough. They liked to do a bit of trading, you know – buckskin jackets and the like. In fact," he added with a reminiscent smile, "one old rascal tried to sell me his squaw."

"A beautiful Indian lady all to yourself?" I asked.

My companion burst out laughing.

"Are you kidding, doctor? He even brought her for me to look at. Beautiful Indian lady! She was a wizened old woman – didn't have a tooth in her head. She must have been eighty if she was a day. She wasn't any bargain, let me tell you!" He continued to chuckle at the memory. "The old son of a gun was quite upset, too, when I told him I wasn't interested. I guess he wanted to get rid of his old woman and make a few bucks at the same time!"

"What were the roads like?" I asked.

"Terrible – at first. Just grass tracks across the prairie. Then we had dirt roads. This road we're on now was just a track across the prairie at one time. It was a day's journey into Calgary, and in the spring the tracks just got churned up into mud.

You could hardly move. So you chose your time to travel if you could. Of course," he went on, "I'm talking about the early days. By the time the twenties came along, Okotoks was real modern, but even before that there were three hotels in the town. But when the railway came through, it went to Calgary and that didn't do our town any good."

We were going over the conduit at Tongue Creek, a few miles north of High River. There is a little dip in the ground there, just beside the road, where the creek, meandering along, is a tiny stream, and I saw my passenger look around him.

"Have you noticed something interesting, Mr. Minue?"

"No. It's just a memory. Would it be a lot of trouble to stop the car for a few minutes?"

I pulled the car into the side of the road. There were a few farmhouses in sight, and the empty road stretched ahead of us. Mr. Minue stood by the roadside looking down at the creek in the shelter of the hollow, and I stood beside him. The only sound was the sighing of the prairie wind.

He didn't speak, and I did not disturb him.

"You've set me to thinking of times gone by," he said, as he walked back to the car. I slipped the car into gear and we moved off.

"Tongue Creek has memories for me," he went on. "When I was young, every summer an Indian and his wife camped there – just down in the hollow beside the creek. I used to have to drive a horse and buggy up to High River once or twice a week, and I'd stop by on my way. Not many people traveled on that trail. I got to know them. They loved tea, I discovered. All Indians loved tea, you know, and I always had some for them. How they looked forward to me coming. I used to stop in on the way back from High River. They would see me a mile or two away on the trail, and the tea'd be ready. Many a cup I had in their tepee – just right back there where we were. It's strange to think of it now, after all these years!"

"What tribe did they belong to?"

"I never knew. They were always alone. They weren't young. I didn't know a word of their language and they didn't know mine. But we got on just fine. And when I'd leave they'd stand together and wave – just like white folks. She was always decently dressed in buckskin but her man just wore a loincloth with a feather stuck in his hair."

I hadn't meant to interrupt him. The words slipped out.

"They were dressed like savages, just sixty years ago?"

The old man looked at me and gently shook his head.

"Savages, doctor? Savages?" he repeated. "I don't know about that. I just know they were nice, respectable people."

Chapter Fourteen

Summer is rodeo time in Alberta, but July means Stampede Week for Calgarians.

During that week, the city worships its western heritage. The Calgary Stampede is called "the greatest outdoor show on earth". There isn't much difference between a stampede and a rodeo, the former being the Canadian version of the American rodeo, but both kinds of events tend to be colorful and exciting for the spectators, dangerous for the contestants.

Calgary's unofficial emblem is the white stetson, and stetsons that have been in cupboards for fifty-one weeks suddenly appear on the streets in thousands. Their wearers – businessmen and shopkeepers the rest of the year – suddenly become cowboys, dressed in western shirts and blue jeans or frontier pants. Cowboys throng the streets, the genuine kind and the drugstore variety, the latter walking perhaps a little uncomfortably in their ceremonial riding boots.

The week begins with the Stampede Parade, headed by some dignitary known for the day as the Grand Marshal. If the marshal is a horseman, and preferably a westerner, he will be in the saddle. Dignitaries who do not ride are accommodated in open cars, but it is not quite the done thing. The crowd will accept the situation, cheer and wave politely, but the public figure who rides a horse for the occasion will be guaranteed a western roar to cheer him on his way.

So, of course, will the Stampede Queen and her two Princesses, and they are always on horseback. The horses will be well worth looking at and so will the girls, chosen for their looks, intelligence, poise and ability to sit well in the saddle.

Then there are the bands. The various regimental bands put on the polished performances one expects. There are sometimes British troops in training on the prairies and their bands, when recognized as being from "the old country", will be given an affectionate cheer.

But perhaps it is the Calgary Highlanders who draw the loudest applause. This is the city's regiment of citizen soldiers, and the sight of the kilts and the skirl of the pipes, raise a roar of approval from the crowd. As do the police pipe band and the clan society bands.

This, however, is not Scotland. It is the Canadian West, a land of immigrants. In the parade are Canadian-Ukrainian dancers, beautiful girls, and athletic young men, and perhaps close behind is a Chinese dragon writhing and weaving its colorful way along the parade route, breathing fire and thunder. There are Danish, Italian, Greek and German folk dancers in native costume, representing all the diverse nationalities that have contributed to this new land, proclaiming their love for the old cultures and their pride in the new.

And the old cultures are well represented. Dignified and impressive with their mahogany complexions and dark eyes surveying the spectators, the Indians ride by, silent, in single file. The buckskin and feathers of the Plains Indians, the Blackfoot, Blood, Sarcee and Stony proclaim their heritage. Their tepees erected in the Indian village at the Stampede grounds add a very authentic touch to the scene.

Then the chuckwagons, those symbols of rangeland culinary art, are driven past, their nonchalant crews waving cheerfully to friends and spectators. The drivers have been busy fellows that morning, cooking pancake breakfasts for the crowds around them.

More bands, students from schools south of the border, Idaho or Wyoming perhaps, the young people marching in that fast shuffle that tends to identify American "marching bands". There is an affiliation between the Canadian and the American West and it is very apparent here today.

And everywhere, children, young people; school bands from Calgary; trick motorcyclists; clowns; and there are visitors from Mexico in sombreros, mounted on gaily caprisoned horses.

It is always a colorful, happy, kaleidoscopic scene. But what claimed our attention at that first stampede parade, as Janet, Catriona, her little friend Mary Rowan and I stood in the crowd, was not so much the color and gaiety of the scene, as the quiet presence of several hundred riders.

They had come in from ranches in the countryside around Okotoks. They rode by on immaculately groomed horses, lariats coiled at the saddles, neatly dressed in western clothes. Here, there was no pretence, no flamboyance. They were the real thing. The ranchers wore their stetsons, tweed jackets and frontier pants as they always did on formal occasions: church, meetings, lunch in Calgary's Palliser Hotel – a favorite dining place for many of them. There were ladies in the saddle in quiet western attire beside their husbands. The ranchers and their wives were unmistakable, and in a quiet way they seemed to me to be saying, "our parents settled this land in the hard times. We began it all."

Beside them rode the ranch hands, younger men and women wearing blue jeans and western shirts – a talkative, cheery bunch, waving to friends in the crowd. Some of them would be competing that week in bronc riding or calf roping contests, taking on the professional cowboys who spend months traveling from one rodeo to the next across North America.

To a man – and woman – these ranchers and their hands were and are experts. That week they would maintain an eagle-eyed criticism of their neighbors' performances as they rode the broncs or were hurtled from them. But they all had farms and ranches to attend to and would not travel far afield that summer to compete. Mostly they would be satisfied to try their skills at local stampedes.

A week previously we had attended a local stampede, the High River Rodeo. We were guests of Dr. and Mrs. Cliff Forsyth, and it was our first visit to such an event. Janet, in her

85

innocence, suggested it might be rather like an English horse show or a county fair and we should pay our hosts the compliment of dressing properly for the occasion. Our appearance taught me that dressing nicely and dressing properly are not one and the same thing.

When we arrived at the Forsyths' door, with Janet in her London finery and me in my business suit, we were met by a doctor and his wife who looked as if they had stepped off the set of a John Wayne movie. At that rodeo we stood out like three sore thumbs, for Miss Gibson was dressed in much the same way as ourselves. Mind you, she had warned us, and we should have listened.

"Daddy!" she had exclaimed in exasperation, "*nobody* dresses like *us* out here. And little girls wear blue jeans to rodeos."

Blue jeans? The idea was quite improper and I refused to consider it. That same week, Janet bought Miss G. her first pair of blue jeans.

I was learning.

The crowd at the rodeo was very western, with "drug store cowboys" conspicuous by their absence. High River is in the heart of Southern Alberta's cattle country, where even little boys and girls can handle horses, and by the time they are teenagers many of them are competing at rodeos.

It was a warm, sunny afternoon when we arrived at the rodeo grounds. There probably were a thousand people there, with "neighbors" who hadn't seen one another for weeks standing talking to one another. In country areas, one's neighbors can live several miles away! There were hundreds more sitting on the bleachers, those long, tiered benches open to sun, wind and rain that line every rodeo ground in Western Canada.

And everywhere, horses. Horses being groomed in the shade of the poplar trees, sweating horses being walked by their riders, horses tethered to posts and trees, horses of every kind and variety being ridden by children and young people.

There were the cowboys, lean-hipped, wiry young men examining harness, readying it for the events. It was like no horse show we had ever attended, and we watched the panorama with fascination. But soon we accompanied our hosts to the bleachers.

86

We had missed some of the events but there was still time, we were told, and we watched with mixed amusement and alarm the bucking broncs hurtling onto the field, rearing and twisting in desperate attempts to rid themselves of their riders. Many of them succeeded, and cowboys would go flying through the air to land on all fours or flat on their faces or backs. It looked as if some of them would never ride again, but within seconds they would be on their feet, ruefully shaking the prairie dust from their clothes, and heading back to the corral.

The climactic ending to the afternoon, however, was to be the chuckwagon races. Chuckwagons are part of the tradition of the West. Those sturdy, four-wheeled wagons followed the great herds of cattle that once were driven for days – and weeks – across the open range to market. Their crews cooked for the cowboys.

Some time towards the beginning of this century, the drivers of two chuckwagons decided to relieve the tedium of their duties by racing their wagons across the open range. So began the rangeland derby. It was a race between wagons pulled by sturdy draft horses, and though it must have been fun, it probably wasn't a very fast race. Chuckwagon races at today's rodeos are fast, dangerous, immensely exciting affairs, run to almost stylized rules. The wagons are pulled by race-horses, four to a team.

The horses, already restless, straining at their bits, stand ready, barely controlled by their drivers, with outriders holding the lead horses' heads. The rangeland stoves sit on the ground at the back of the wagons, with two more of the crew crouched over each stove, tense, ready to throw them into the wagons at the drop of the rodeo marshal's hat. It is no easy task to accomplish, for they must hold their horses too, and they, in turn, affected by the excitement around them, are sweating and restless.

Suddenly the marshal, assured that the contestants are properly in position, drops his stetson and there is a roar, "They're off!" from the spectators and the race is on. The stoves must be thrown into the wagons or the delinquent crew is disqualified. But once begun there is little that can be done to check the power and speed of the animals.

The stoves are in. The wagons circle the barrels. Only the

skill of the drivers can prevent collisions. Then on to the circuit in a mad rush, jockeying for position. The outriders have flung themselves onto their horses and streak to catch up with their wagon. Stetsons fly off. Dust rises in clouds. The yells of drivers urging on their teams are lost in the roar of the crowd, on its feet now. The wagons, three at a time, thunder past, round the bend and into the straight. Suddenly the race is over. The dust drifts along the empty track as the spectators wait, impatiently, for the next race.

We had watched two races and I was filled with admiration for the daring skill of the drivers, the horsemanship of the outriders. Then things went wrong.

It was the final event of the day. Three wagons thundered onto the track, neck and neck, as they reached the bleachers. A wagon slewed to one side, tilted over and began to fall. Wheels touched. Suddenly a driver was catapulted forward, thrown into the air and fell under the galloping animals. The second driver, oblivious at first to what had happened, raced on, the driverless team just behind him. The wagon that had fallen was dragged along the track with the driver, by some miracle, still hanging on to the reins, hauling the horses to a stop.

But an inert body lay on the track just in front of us. Instinctively Cliff and I vaulted the railing together and ran to him. Blood, I remember, was trickling from his ear.

Dr. Forsyth said urgently, "Just get him off the track. Those runaways'll be on top of us in seconds."

The crowd, wildly enthusiastic before, was deadly quiet. Men were on the track now, running toward the curve, toward the runaways. We lifted our patient to safety just as the driverless horses came tearing round the bend. They didn't get very far. It took courage for men to hurl themselves at them, seize their harness and drag them by brute force and skill to a halt. But they did it, and calmed the trembling animals as they stood beside them, watching the scene further down the track where a smashed wagon lay on its side and horses, entangled in their harness, struggled and kicked, with men working feverishly to free them.

Soon the ambulance was beside us. Carefully we lifted the unconscious driver onto a stretcher. The other driver, who had hauled his overturned wagon to a halt, was persuaded to accompany us, and limping badly, he too climbed into the ambulance.

The hospital had been notified of the accident and the emergency room readied. The driver who had accompanied us insisted that he could wait and we turned our attention to the youth who lay unconscious on the stretcher. He had broken ribs, a fractured skull, and probably hemorrhage into the brain, we thought.

Dr. Forsyth took charge, telephoned a neurosurgeon in Calgary, did all he could do at a small hospital in such a case, and speedily our patient was on his way to Calgary's General Hospital for the specialized care he desperately needed.

The second driver also required treatment. He had broken ribs and a badly wrenched knee, already swollen, but he made light of his injuries, and since he lived in the area, I arranged to see him in our kitchen-office in several days' time. He was a tough-looking, stocky man in his forties, not much taller than myself, dressed in blue jeans and a colorful western shirt. As I examined him, he told me that one of the horses had broken a leg in the accident and had to be destroyed.

"I'm sorry to hear that," I said, sympathetically. His only reply was a nod. It was easy to see that he was upset. However tough he might be physically, I thought, his employer wasn't likely to be too happy about that horse, but I said nothing and he went away.

Dr. Forsyth's assessment had been correct in the case of the young driver who had been trampled. He lay in a coma, his outlook far from promising.

As he had said he would, my patient presented himself in Okotoks in a few days' time so that I could check his knee and chest. He was wearing the same clothes, old blue jeans, bleached and patched, well-worn cowboy boots and the same shirt, now neatly laundered.

"I'm sorry about that accident," I said, as I probed, pushed and flexed his knee, "but I suppose you're lucky. It could have been a lot worse."

"I guess," was his laconic reply. "What's your bill, doc?"

"Oh, there won't be any bill," I replied, commiseratingly. "I had a great afternoon, and I should think your boss wasn't too pleased about that horse. So we'll forget the bill."

"No we won't," said my unsmiling visitor. "And what's this about 'my boss'? I *am* the boss. I own that outfit. I own two thousand acres of land, so I don't need any charity from anybody – or sympathy," he added. "So just tell me your bill, doctor, and I'll be on my way."

It was another lesson. I never again judged a man's position by his looks, dress, accent or appearance. We had come to a different culture.

Our young patient lay in a coma for days, but a year later he was back in the saddle and then, miraculously or foolhardily, whichever way you care to look at it, he was back in the driver's seat of a chuckwagon!

Chapter
Fifteen

The first doctors to come to Alberta were still remembered by many of the older people we knew. To some, they were almost revered, even legendary figures. At the turn of the century they had been men on their own in that vast, empty land, tackling whatever surgery they had to, sometimes heroically, thus starting the tradition of the general practitioner surgeon.

Many of them were well trained and had studied at the great medical centers of Europe. Returning to Canada after their years at Edinburgh or Vienna, they had settled in the West, and what towers of strength they must have been to settlers on the almost trackless plains of those early days.

They were the original "horse and buggy doctors". There were some very strong men among them, and I heard stories of how, in the depths of winter, they would keep two teams of horses working in rotation. Muffled in buffalo robes and coats, in open sleighs, they made their lonely and often hazardous rounds, ministering to the sick in one farmhouse, and perhaps operating in another, with the patient on the kitchen table. It took great strength of character for caring physicians to undertake such work, with perhaps more tragedies than triumphs in those days before modern drugs and hospitals.

In summer, however, in the horse-drawn "buggies" that gave them their nickname, they must have had time to enjoy the crisp, early-morning prairie air, to bask in the sunshine and glory in the magnificence of the western sky. And they must have had time to philosophize.

But the horse and buggy doctors have vanished into the mists of antiquity, their legacy a tradition of humanitarianism and a ready acceptance of the general practitioner surgeon.

In 1901, when Calgary's population was a few thousand, the "city" consisted of clapboard houses and wooden sidewalks. The first hospital was a small house, with mostly general practitioners doing whatever medicine and surgery had to be done.

By 1961, the city had a population of just under 250,000 and had highly specialized medical and surgical facilities, while ten years later, with a population of 400,000 and on its way to becoming a metropolis, it had its own medical school.

Perhaps only fifteen percent of Alberta's population now live in the country and small towns, and one needs only to drive along prairie roads, past one deserted farmhouse after another, through once flourishing villages standing dilapidated and half forsaken, to realize that the population shift from the countryside to the city is probably irreversible. Consequently some "one doctor towns" will eventually lose their elderly physicians and they will not be replaced.

But some small centers are growing, their hospitals and medical staffs being enlarged. Sizable hospitals with modern facilities attract specialists, and towns that twenty or thirty years ago were serviced by general practitioners often have a surgeon or two on the staff today.

I have never forgotten how, when I was a medical student, Professor Sir Archibald Young, Regius professor of surgery at Glasgow, once said to several of us, "In your lives you will be called upon to make decisions and take action that may cause you torment of spirit, and others grief. Never have regrets if, in conscience, you have done the right thing."

There is seldom a need for such heroic decisions today, as communications and technology have vastly improved patients' chances of survival. There are more, and better roads. The newer hospitals in North America have helicopter pads in the grounds, and emergency cases requiring specialized care can be flown from small hospitals to large ones rapidly and smoothly, with nurses or doctors in attendance during the flight. It is all becoming very modern and safe compared to those days of twenty or thirty years ago.

Alberta, with its newborn death rate of 7.5 per 100,000 live births is one of the safest places in the world in which to have a baby. This is the result of careful planning as well as the splendid advances in technology that allow possible complications to be foreseen, and steps taken to avoid them. Where complications may arise, mothers-to-be are nowadays referred to specialized centers. Where surgery is concerned, the College of Physicians and Surgeons maintains a careful watch over the records and activities of operators.

But thirty years ago, the local hospital boards usually had the final say as to who might do what in surgery. Lax boards might not care very much about their responsibilities in policing activities within the hospital, and gullible ones could be "taken in" by smooth-talking physicians, or by doctors who mistakenly thought they were God's gift (however poorly trained) to surgery.

I was lucky. The Board at High River was knowledgeable. I worked with colleagues who recognized my surgical limitations and they took the trouble to teach me.

They were all "g.p. surgeons." The older men accepted surgery as part of their way of life. They were still part of the tradition engendered by the harsh and lonely conditions of their young days, and the traditions left by those splendid men, the horse and buggy doctors of the prairies. Some of them had had extensive training, although few of them had any desire to be specialists. What they did, they did well. Although my own surgical skills were limited, I admired their all-round competence, and I saw very few avoidable catastrophes. I was fortunate to have such men as colleagues and teachers.

Within a couple of weeks I was happily assisting at operations, being coached in reading X-ray films, looking down microscopes at blood slides, watching and learning.

Eventually, I became a useful member of the operating room team, but Canada's medical services were beginning to attract the attention of politicians and there were calls for change. One suggestion made was that all surgery should be done in centralized hospitals by fully qualified specialists. Logically, it was said, patients would receive better care there.

On the face of it, it was a commendable idea. When we are sick, we all want the best care we can get. But it was an impractical proposal. How could emergency cases be transferred in blizzard conditions? The ferocity of the prairie blizzards has to be experienced to be appreciated. Desirable, impractical or not, the suggestion prompted a good deal of acrimonious discussion among my colleagues, some of whom, competent surgeons despite their lack of specialist certificates, resented the suggestion that the care they gave their patients might not be good enough.

In a sense, I was a bystander, for surgery was something I could take or leave, even though years had passed and I could tackle emergencies capably enough. But most of the surgery in our practice was referred either to the men I worked with at High River, or to specialists in Calgary.

Local people had pride in their hospitals, and a loyalty to their own doctors. They often had to be persuaded that some other physician or surgeon should even be consulted, let alone asked to operate on them. It was all part of the tradition of prairie medicine.

"Why can't you do it, doc?" they'd say. "If I trust you, isn't that enough?"

Then there was the question of convenience. Farmers don't like taking time off work, especially during summer and fall, and they want to be close to home, where they can still direct their affairs. Distant hospitals meant a lack of communication and fewer visitors. And in "their hospitals" there was often a warmth, a sense of "belonging" that was sometimes lacking in the coolly impersonal atmosphere of large institutions.

In Okotoks, night calls tended to come in runs, but they seemed to slacken off in bad weather. It had been snowing heavily earlier that day, but now the skies were cloudless. The stars in their myriads glittered in the purple-blue of the heavens and the moonglow cast every snowbank into soft relief. It was beautiful outside. But it was cold, perhaps thirty below, and no weather to be out on lonely roads.

Country folk, knowing the dangers that lie in such cold, enthralling beauty, avoided calling us in such weather if they could, and we expected a peaceful night.

"You'd better check the roads, just in case," said Janet, as we sipped a late night coffee.

So I rang the Mounted Police barracks.

"The main roads have been plowed out. Most of the sideroads are blocked. The road between here and High River is clear, doc," said my young friend, adding cheerfully, "so if you're thinking of delivering a baby tonight you've got a clear run up to the hospital."

"Not tonight, Josephine," I replied, and went to bed.

It was one o'clock in the morning when the telephone rang and the voice at the other end said,

"It's the hospital here. One moment please," followed almost instantly by one of my colleagues saying,

"Can you get up here – *fast*?"

"Yes. The road's been plowed out."

"Then don't ask questions! Just move."

I threw myself into the jersey, slacks, socks, snowboots, fur-lined parka, hat and gloves that were always at hand, and ran for the car. Fifteen miles flew by and I slammed on my brakes as I raced into the hospital yard.

A nurse, waiting for me, stood inside the main door. She hurried along the corridor beside me.

"I'm to tell you to get into the O.R. as fast as you can, doctor. I've laid your things out for you."

"What's wrong?"

"A lady has been brought in from twenty miles out. It's taken them two hours to get her here through drifts, even with the neighbors helping. She's in awful shape. It's a ruptured ectopic."

An ectopic or tubal pregnancy occurs when the fertilized human ovum becomes implanted, not in the womb, where it should be, but in the tube leading to the womb. Such an abnormality is comparatively uncommon, occurring in about one in two hundred pregnancies. It is also highly dangerous and must be dealt with surgically. Our patient had been confused by her symptoms. Were the recent pains in her abdomen simply "stomach flu?" Why had she had a short period? If she was pregnant, as she had thought, it was too early to see any doctor. Was she pregnant at all, she wondered? Suddenly late that night she had experienced acute tearing pain in her abdomen and had collapsed. Whatever it was, she needed help quickly and so her nerve-wracking journey to the hospital had begun.

Their truck became stuck in snowdrifts. Neighboring farmers turned out their tractors, hauled the truck through one drift after another. A farmer in another tractor went ahead of them, clearing the road as best he could. When she reached the hospital, internal bleeding from the ruptured ovarian tube had reached catastrophic proportions and Mrs. James, our patient, was barely conscious.

Quickly I changed and hurried into the operating room. All was bustle. Nurses, gowned and masked, were hurrying about their tasks, while the surgeon stood ready, quietly giving instructions. The patient, as pale as a ghost, lay on the operating table.

I strode over to my colleague.

"What d'you want me to do?" I quietly asked, "assist or give the anesthetic?"

"You're first here," he replied. "Anesthetize her. We've got to go ahead. McCaulay's on his way. He'll assist when he gets here. I've got a drip going," he added, "and what a job it was to find a vein. She's awfully flat."

"I can see that," I replied grimly as I made for the anesthetist's equipment. It had been checked and was ready for instant use. One glance at the woman's deathly white face convinced me of the disastrous emergency that confronted us.

The abdomen was swollen. She was bleeding internally and

heavily. Thankfully, the intravenous drip was running freely, but the patient's blood pressure barely registered. My colleague sensed my thoughts.

"We can't wait," he said quietly. "There's more blood on the way from Calgary. The Mounties are bringing it. We have to get started, whatever happens."

As I began to administer the anesthetic, I wondered if she would die on the table. Only once or twice in my life have I had reason to fear this, and I felt fear now, but the capacity of the human body to withstand great damage has always interested and puzzled me. Mrs. James, despite the appearance of being *in extremis*, proceeded to astound me. Strangely it was an easy anesthetic to give.

Quickly she was "asleep" and as quickly my colleague was at work. The abdomen was opened. Blood seemed to be everywhere. It was scooped out in clotted handfuls and cast into the waiting sterile basins, held ready by nurses. The only sounds to be heard were quiet requests for instruments.

"How's she doing at your end?" the surgeon asked me.

"She amazes me. The blood pressure's even rising."

"Good. As soon as I can see where the bleeding's coming from I'll have it stopped and we'll be home free – I hope," replied my friend, grimly.

Dr. McCaulay had joined us; he stopped for a moment, his head to one side.

"Listen!" he said, "I hear the police car siren – it's a long way off, but surely it's the blood."

Suddenly the surgeon looked up.

"Got it!" he said in triumph. "She won't bleed any more tonight. Count sponges. Let's get the abdomen closed!"

Blood-soaked swabs were laid out, counted and recounted; instruments checked. The blood arrived. The anesthetic was discontinued. Our charge was lifted onto the operating room trolley and taken to the recovery room, where I stood by.

"How's she doing?" asked my colleagues when I returned.

"Just fine," I replied. "I guess we were lucky."

"She was, you mean," was the reply. "Just suppose she had to be taken to Calgary tonight for surgery. She wouldn't have made it ten miles down the road. She'd have died. Better g.p. surgeons and anesthetists than none at all, my friend."

It was true. Even with our limited resources and training, we had saved a life. It was a little drama that over the years has been repeated time and time again in North America's country hospitals.

But forces for change are often inexorable. The horse and buggy doctor is only a memory, and before too many years have passed, the g.p. surgeon, even on the prairies, will follow him.

Chapter Sixteen

There is a story told of the MacNeils who, in ancient times, ruled over Bara, a small, lonely island off the west coast of Scotland. They were a warlike lot, though a small clan, and wisely had built themselves a castle – a small castle, ruled over by their chief, "The MacNeil of Bara".

The MacNeil, like most of his clansmen, had, as they say in Scotland, "a decent conceit of himself", and every evening, before dinner, his piper would appear on the castle battlements, delighting his audience with the fervor of his piping. The performance completed, the piper would announce to a listening world that: "The MacNeil of Bara is about to dine".

Later the piper would reappear on the battlements, to declare in his Scotch Gaelic that "The MacNeil has dined, and now the princes of the world may eat." The story is probably apocryphal.

In rather the same kind of vein, the Calgary Stampede hosts the World Championship chuckwagon races. It doesn't matter that practically all the competing wagons come from nearby small towns such as Innisfail, Blackie and Airdrie. There may have been a few entrants over the years from such international centers as Blackfoot, Montana, and Buffalo, Wyoming, too, but none I have noticed from Salzburg, Edinburgh or Paris.

There is nothing apocryphal about the history of Calgary's chuckwagon races. Apocalyptic would be a more appropriate word, I used to think, as I watched that mess of men, horses, and trucks hurtle around the track. It constantly amazes me that so few serious accidents do occur.

Although my friendship with Jack Sparrow was growing, somehow I did not associate him with an enthusiasm for chuckwagon races, and was taken aback when he arrived at our door one morning to say that he had obtained three extra seats on the bleachers and would we accompany his wife and himself to the finals.

"I've got a personal interest in this," he explained. "I've a horse running in the fourth heat and I've got to be there. It's the lead horse d'you see, and," he added, "I intend to see it take that wagon to victory."

The climactic ending to the stampede, the finals of the chuck-wagon races, always took place on a Saturday night, and we traveled in Jack's car. The back seat looked very respectable. It had been cleared of all impediments such as ropes, spades, and gasoline cans. I sat in state in the front seat, which was just as well, since I could hang on to the door. Janet and Catriona sat in the back with Molly Sparrow.

The door, as Jack put it, still "had an abominable habit of flying open for no reason at all."

We arrived at the Stampede grounds in time to join the crowds that were already packing the benches. The world about us, cheerful and colorful, was worth watching. There wasn't a cloud in the sky and although the sun was moving toward the horizon, the dry evening air was warm.

Nor was the air the only dry thing. Alberta was a "dry" province. The laws regarding liquor were strict. Wine could not be consumed with hotel meals. The public possession of liquor was frowned upon, both legally and morally. If the rules were seldom flouted, they were frequently circumvented.

"Would the mayor return to the cloakroom at once," roared the announcer over the public address system. "Your worship, your attaché case is leaking."

It was an old chestnut, but the crowd loved it, showed its amused approval and settled down for the first race.

An Indian passed us. He was a big husky fellow, dressed in blue jeans, wearing a black stetson with a feather stuck in the hat band. With his mahogany complexion, black braids, aquiline nose and dark eyes, he was an imposing looking man. But he was drunk.

Jack Sparrow saw me watching him and said, "he's either Blackfoot or Stony, I'd say, in for the week from the concentration camp."

"Concentration camp?"

"His reserve. It wasn't the Germans that invented concentration camps, you know. It was us. During the Boer War the British moved thousands of Boer women and children into what they even called concentration camps. Thousands died. They weren't killed deliberately, of course. They died of infectious diseases. We were a bit more polite about it in Canada. We moved the Indians into reserves. We don't kill them, either. We just don't give a damn."

I looked at my companion. His face was impassive, but I felt his sympathy for the Indian making his unsteady way towards the infield.

"Some of these fellows spend the summers going from one rodeo to another," he went on. "They live for horses, yet half of them neglect them when they've got them. They'll compete if they can, but there's too much drinking goes on with a lot of them, and they land in jail."

"What's the answer?" I asked.

"Don't ask me!" was the reply. "Ask the politicians. Education's one answer, but the old chiefs don't want to see the kids educated like white men. Throw them out of the reserves. Make them fend for themselves, that's another possibility. But you see, we no more understand them than they understand us. We've destroyed whatever culture they had. They're lost."

"Look at him," he went on, nodding toward the Indian. "I bet he doesn't do a stroke of work. He's living on government handouts in a world he can't compete in. There goes the end result of the Welfare State."

I looked at Jack, surprised once again by the incisiveness of his comments. Like several Albertans I had talked to, he had compassion for the native peoples, although this compassion was often mixed with impatience.

The final heats began. The world championship for that year was to be decided that evening and the crowd's expectant excitement grew.

Wagons were appearing in the infield now, and were quietly circling the upturned barrels they must soon round at the start of each race. We could see other teams outside the arena, where drivers were walking their teams in readiness for their heat, outriders were trotting or cantering their horses, men were checking harness.

Suddenly everything was ready. The first race was about to begin. The wagons were in place, the drivers poised, tense, waiting for the ring marshal to canter past and throw his hat to the ground, in the time-honored style.

The hat was down. They were off. Stoves were thrown in; the wagons swung round the barrels, neck and neck. They were on the track. Horses were going like the wind; outriders frantically urged their mounts to greater speed. Dust rose in clouds, and as the whole hurtling mass rounded the bend and came thundering down the straight in front of the grandstand, the crowd was on its feet, roaring encouragement. Suddenly, the race was over. The winner would appear later in the final.

Soon heat three was over, and I reminded Jack to point out his horse to me when it appeared in the infield. He nodded, then suddenly exclaimed,

"There he is! The lead horse in the Buckley outfit!"

Each chuckwagon is a miniature covered wagon, the canvas showing the name of its sponsor or owner and I could easily see Jack Sparrow's horse.

"Watch this!" he said. "That horse is going to take that wagon to the championship tonight. Lars Porsena – a wonderful horse, I tell you."

"Lars Porsena?" I echoed in disbelief. "That's the name of your horse?"

"What's wrong with that?" our host demanded to know. "A noble animal deserves a noble name."

100

"But Lars Porsena! He was a character in Macaulay's *Lays of Ancient Rome*."

"Indeed he was," replied my friend. "Lars Porsena was the bravest of them all."

There was some activity in the infield. Teams were getting into place and several flighty horses were giving trouble to their drivers. But not Lars Porsena. He stood there, as steady as a rock.

Jack stood on his feet then, and amidst cries of "Shut up!" and "Siddown!" he declaimed:

> Lars Porsena of Clusium,
> By the nine gods he swore,
> That the great house of Tarquin,
> Should suffer wrong no more.
>
> By the nine gods he swore it,
> And named a trysting day,
> And bade his messengers ride forth,
> East and West and South and North,
> To summon his array.

A particularly loud bellow to "Shut up, you, and sit down," from a gentleman immediately behind us caused a short interruption in the flow of eloquence.

Turning round and surveying his interrupter with stony-faced dignity, our host said quietly,

"When I'm good and ready," then recited the lines:

> Oh Tiber! father Tiber,
> To whom the Romans pray,
> A Roman's life, a Roman's arms,
> Take them in charge this day!

"Thank you," he said with a nod to the man behind, then sat down.

The race began. Round the barrels and off, with Lars Porsena in the lead, his mane flowing in the wind. On to the track in a melee of flying hooves and wheels.

101

"Just look at him," said Jack Sparrow. "Look at him go!"

But what was this? A team was gaining on the Buckley outfit. Slowly it pulled alongside, neck and neck – then past. Lars Porsena was in second place. On! Lars Porsena, on! Remember your heritage!

"Goddam," Jack said. "It's the driver's fault. Get on, Porsena!" he bawled as if his voice alone would urge his protégé to victory.

But, alas, it was not to be. Lars Porsena, like Casey, that other illustrious literary figure, had struck out.

Jack Sparrow was somewhat peeved.

He intended, he said, to have a word with the driver, and invited me to go with him. I at first declined the invitation, but on his urging, I accompanied him.

We went no further than the cavernous vaults underneath the grandstand. There, my friend, having satisfied himself that no members of the Calgary police force were nearby, reached into his hip pocket and produced the whisky flask I had seen once before. He was raising the flask to his mouth when he stopped and proffered it to me.

"We need some anesthetic, you and me," he said, "so help yourself," adding once again, "goddam! Lars Porsena should've won, y'know; it was the driver's fault, and when I see him . . ."

On the way home, Janet, who loves poetry, complimented our host on his knowledge, and asked him if he knew much of Burns' work.

"A great poet, but a weak man," said Jack, before launching into a dissertation on Burns that would have done credit to a university lecturer, and soon Janet and he were taking turns in reciting their favorite poems.

Lars Porsena's defeat and disgrace had been forgotten. We had had a wonderful time. Little Miss Gibson tumbled into bed and was fast asleep in seconds.

And I, as we prepared for bed, said to my better half,

"D'you remember old Ponsonby in Hull who told me I'd find no 'character' out west, no culture, nobody to talk to? NO CHARACTER!!"

Chapter
Seventeen

The summer of 1955 was beautiful, with dry, warm days and cool nights. Day after day the sun shone down from an azure sky, undisturbed by a single trespassing cloud. The land, from the rolling prairies in the east to the sloping foothills in the west was as green as any field in verdant Ireland. It was an idyllic existence for us and would remain so for months to come.

One afternoon in September, I was driving to High River to see a patient, when I saw a small, dumpy figure trudging in the same direction. She was walking in the ditch, not a shallow trench like those that line British roads, but a prairie ditch, feet deep and wide enough to accommodate a truck. Over the winter months those ditches are gradually filled to the brim by the hard snow of the western plains. In summer they grow lush and green, and walking in the ditch is much more pleasant than tramping along roads in the dusty wake of passing cars.

She was not a young woman. Dressed in a black skirt and a nondescript woolen pullover, a black beret placed squarely over her dark hair, and carrying a brown leather handbag, she trudged steadily toward town, paying not the slightest attention to my car as it passed.

And yet, my old car was the only one in sight for miles ahead or behind. The nearest farmhouse, well back from the road, was a mile away, and she had a long way to go if High River was her goal.

Curiously, I watched her in my rearview mirror after I had passed. Albertans, especially country folk, are not given to walking for idle pleasure. She was trudging forward, steadily, purposefully. She was of indeterminate age, fifty perhaps, maybe sixty, and it was hot for the time of year and not the best of days to be walking in the full glare of the sun.

I pulled the car over to the side of the road, stopped and waited. She was a hundred or two yards behind me at that point, but soon drew abreast of the car. She gave me a passing glance and would undoubtedly have kept on walking.

"I'm going to High River. Can I give you a lift?"

She looked at me, did not reply, changed direction, climbed up the steep bank of the ditch and without a word took the passenger seat. I held the door open for her, closed it, walked round to the driver's seat and started the engine.

"It's a beautiful day, isn't it?"

Apparently she hadn't heard me. She stared straight ahead, and I gave up any attempt at polite conversation. She could be deaf, I thought, or she could be an immigrant like myself, but perhaps one who didn't have a word of English.

Suddenly I felt sorry for her. Already Canada was "home" to us, but our ability to speak English gave us a tremendous advantage over poor souls like this, whose difficulties must be enormous, I thought. Wordlessly we reached the outskirts of High River, round the only bend on that long stretch of road, past the first wooden houses, their white paint reflecting the sun's rays.

"Where," I asked slowly, "do you wish to go?"

"Bradley's," she replied in a low voice. At least she wasn't deaf.

I knew Bradley's Western Store. It would have been almost impossible for a wide-eyed, innocent Britisher like me to miss it. The windows were full of stetsons, blue jeans, cowboy boots and usually a saddle or two. A prominent notice challenged the locals:

"Men," it said, "buy your saddles on credit."

I stopped the car at Bradley's door. My passenger alighted, held the car door open, looked me straight in the eye and said in an astoundingly beautiful voice, "What's your name?"

"Gibson," I replied, agape.

"Where do you come from?"

"Okotoks."

"Couldn't you have done better for yourself than pick up an old broad like me?"

As the last mellifluous notes of her voice faded, she tramped into the shop and disappeared from view.

It was her voice that amazed me, but her appearance perplexed me. Stout, unsmiling, dressed in dowdy black, she might have been a peasant woman. But that voice proclaimed education, breeding, and as I told Janet later that evening, there "was something about her". Somehow, she was not the kind of person you would easily forget.

Canada, we agreed once again, really was a land of surprises.

Our Skye Glen schoolhouse was by now an adequate office and with the help of a part-time receptionist, we felt we were once again entering the mainstream of medical practice, at least the mainstream for rural Alberta.

One afternoon, a week after my encounter with this strange woman, I was sitting at my desk. Our receptionist was guarding the empty waiting room. We were not busy. I had four patients booked for that afternoon. Janet had none, and so Catriona and she were gathering wild flowers on the hill behind our house. Our receptionist quietly opened the door and slipped into my office. For a normally very composed young lady, she looked rather startled.

"There's a lady out there to see you," she said, adding in a significant whisper, "and is she ever *different!*"

The visitor was ushered in. It was my passenger of the week before. She took in her surroundings with one sweeping inspection. The furniture was rapidly appraised and no doubt classified as secondhand. The colored prints on the wall were glanced at and so was the framed certificate stating that I was qualified to practise medicine in Alberta. Finally I was inspected.

"Good afternoon, doctor. You didn't tell me your occupation when we met."

"No, er, it didn't seem necessary."

"I see. Are you any good as a doctor?" she asked in that beautiful modulated voice. I didn't know whether to bridle or smile. The question had been asked matter-of-factly but with detached courtesy and she stood there, her eyes on my face, waiting for my reply.

"I try to be."

"That is no answer. Any fool can *try* to be. I asked if you are a *good* doctor?"

"I believe I'm a good doctor."

"Are you as good as Tommy Horder?"

I tried to control the sudden slackening in my jaw muscles.
Tommy Horder? I thought. *The* Tommy Horder? Lord Hor-

der. England's most famous specialist and doctor to the Royal family? *That* Tommy Horder?

"No," I replied with caution, "I don't think I could claim to be in the same class as Lord Horder."

"Why not? Don't disparage yourself. Tommy Horder is mortal, and God knows fallible like all of us. He's very human. You may be a *very* good doctor. Do you know Lord Horder?"

Strangely enough I had met him several times, had had dinner with him and found him to be a blunt, self-assured yet modest and humorous man. Unlike some of his fellow physicians from Harley Street, there was nothing god-like about him. My visitor knew Lord Horder probably a great deal better than I did, I thought, and politely I hinted that such might be the case.

"Tommy was my doctor when I lived in London. He was also my friend. I have decided that you shall be my doctor," she announced imperiously.

"Er-er, thank you," I stammered, "that's very good of you . . ."

I had made a mistake.

"There's nothing good about it," she corrected me. "I hope I may never require your services."

"Er – I'm afraid I don't know your name?"

"Odette."

"Odette, er, yes . . .?" I noticed she wasn't wearing a wedding ring.

"Odette de Foras."

"Thank you. It's very nice to meet you, Miss de Foras . . ."

"I am Odette, Countess de Foras," she corrected me.

I stared at my "peasant woman" of the week before, thunderstruck at this change in the situation. I was to learn more about her within the next few days, and even more in the next twenty-three years, with the lady as our patient – often a difficult, but never a dull patient.

Odette's father, the Count de Foras, had left France for Southern Alberta in the early days of settlement. He probably found himself socially at home in the company of some of his fellow pioneers, many of whom were moneyed Englishmen. They could afford to live in considerable style, having brought butlers and maids from the old country as well as the mistaken belief that they could live in Western Canada like landed ger*ry, for land was cheap. Alas, there were no peasants there willing to work for wages. There were only other settlers, independent men, working hard to clear their own land.

Before long, some of the well-to-do, realizing their mistake, had gone home. Others stayed on, became farmers or ranchers, kept polo ponies on the side, imported good livestock and made solid contributions to their new homeland.

Count de Foras was never a wealthy man, despite his highly acceptable social background. But there were immensely wealthy men in Alberta, and one of those was Pat Burns, an immigrant Irishman who by sheer brains and determination had become one of Western Canada's first cattle barons. His legendary success as a cattleman has sometimes dimmed his other attributes, for Burns, a Canadian by adoption, was a quiet, generous philanthropist.

Calgary was a pioneer town of six thousand people in the early 1900s. Burns heard Odette sing at some local concert. She was then a young girl and the cattleman was deeply impressed by the beauty of her voice. Burns, so the story goes, persuaded the Count to send his daughter to Italy for formal training as a singer.

Odette became famous. She sang in London's Royal Opera House before royalty, was acclaimed and befriended by conductors as famous as Bruno Walter. Before she reached the heights of fame that seemed to lie just before her, she suddenly retired, vowed she would never sing in public again and returned to the family farm at High River, to live there alone, and to farm the land. When she relented, as she did on one or two rare occasions, or sang for friends, she had the voice of an angel.

She had a great affection for young people, and was an incisive judge of character. Where she saw talent, skill and intelligence in youngsters, she encouraged it forcefully and sometimes her approach to young people was alarming in its directness. Catriona and Mary she especially terrified. That was all right. Sometimes she terrified me too.

This was the woman who was watching me now, as I tried to appear unsurprised at this announcement of her title.

"I am known as Odette," she went on. "Simply Odette. My friends sometimes call me Tiger. *You* may call me Tiger."

She bowed graciously, turned and opened the door to leave. Then she looked back at me.

"If you wish to be formal," she said, "you may call me Madame de Foras. But," with that mellifluous voice rising an octave or two, "*Never* for Christ's sake, call me *Miss* de Foras."

Many years later, when I was a university teacher of medicine, Odette remained my patient. I saw patients on two afternoons of each week, and before too long my sessions became "Okotoks days" to the nurses. The waiting area was filled with stetson-hatted men and their wives in from the country; the place abuzz with talk of wheat and cattle, and I enjoyed seeing old friends.

Odette always had refused to discuss her age. She disclosed it to no one. Age, she said emphatically, was a matter of resilience of mind. She was, I suspected, well on the wrong side of seventy when one day she arrived at my office door.

I took her to lunch in the Medical School Mall, a democratic affair with a self-service cafeteria where teachers and students often sit together. Odette and I sat at a small table. The place was crowded. There was a great deal of coming and going and much talk.

Suddenly Odette said, "I shall sing."

She rose to her feet, placed one hand upon the other and sang Schubert's *Ave Maria*. Her voice was still magnificent. There was a sudden hush as the high notes filled that great hall. It was the voice, not of an old lady whose life was nearing its end, but of a young girl, full of joy and hope.

Half embarrassed, I looked about me, at my colleagues, the students and the singer. All eyes were fastened on that dumpy little figure as she stood there, pouring out her soul in that beautiful song. There was absolute stillness around me, and when she finished there was a roar of delight from her listeners. They rose to their feet, clapped thunderously and shouted for more.

But Odette bowed, bowed again and sat down. When we finished lunch, we strolled back to my office. There she ferreted around in that bag she always carried, produced a photograph and said, "I have brought you a memento."

The photograph was of a poised, curvaceous young woman in court dress and wearing a tiara.

"Myself," said Odette, "as Tosca."

I was still looking at the photograph when she said,

"If you had known me then – would you have kissed me?"

"I should say so!"

"Well then," said the lady, "you may do so now."

And I did.

Chapter Eighteen

I hadn't seen much of Jack Sparrow since the day I gouged his tooth out – but I'd learned a lot about him.

If his name was Shakespearean, the man himself was an Elizabethan. He would have made a splendid buccaneer. He also had a complex and brilliant mind, with a knowledge of the Law that was encyclopedic. The subject fascinated him, just as it challenged him, for Jack Sparrow was a born intellectual.

He was almost totally self-educated. At the age of sixteen he was an infantryman in France during the Great War. He had fought at Vimy Ridge, been badly wounded at Passchendaele, had captured a German brigade staff single-handed and twice won the Military Medal. To the men who had fought with him (and there were several of them still living in Okotoks), Sparrow was a legendary figure.

They told me that he had several times done enough to win the Victoria Cross, for in the hell of trench warfare when others faltered, Sparrow had rallied them and led them forward. His seemed to be a charmed life. Time and time again he had volunteered for deadly work. He was a formidable sniper. But, they'd say, with the reminiscent grins of old soldiers, Jack never retained his newly won stripes for any length of time, and they'd recall some of his exploits, none of them supportive of "good order and discipline".

He had routed more than the enemy, too, his old comrades told me. In later years he'd appear in magistrates' courts on behalf of friends and conduct their cases. He seldom lost one. In one instance he appeared on his own behalf in one of the higher courts of Alberta. Mr. Sparrow had been caught speeding – or to put it in more legalistic terms, he had been caught *allegedly* speeding and issued with a ticket for the offence. He refused to pay. Outraged at the effrontery and the injustice of such an arbitrary decision, Jack Sparrow appealed the magistrate's decision and found himself in the High Court. There was something about the situation that would have appealed to Gilbert and Sullivan.

It became a celebrated case at the time, for His Lordship took the strongest exception to Mr. Sparrow, a mere landscape gardener, appearing on his own behalf. Where, he wanted to know, was Mr. Sparrow's counsel? It was neither proper nor wise, advised the judge, whose peppery temper was well known, that Mr. Sparrow should be unrepresented by legal counsel. Mr. Sparrow, never a man to be intimidated, disagreed. His Lordship, showing signs of rising irritability, announced that he would not allow him to conduct the case. Mr. Sparrow felt quite capable of giving a good account of himself. There was a heated discussion. Finally His Lordship snapped,

"No, y'can't do it. I won't allow it, and that's that!"

"And why not, m'lord?" Mr. Sparrow had asked silkily.

"Why not?" roared the exasperated judge, "I'll tell you why not. Because y' don't belong to the lawyers' union. That's why not." Whereupon Mr. Sparrow, who as usual had done his homework, produced the legislation that gave the citizen the right to appear, even in one of the most exalted courts of law in Alberta, on his own behalf.

The judge, fuming, capitulated. Sparrow put up a brilliant defence, won the case and earned the public congratulations of a judge whose irascibility and reluctance had been won over by this layman's ability.

Not that Jack won all his battles.

He was not the most punctilious of drivers. Furthermore his mechanical skills were minimal. His car, an ancient and dilapidated Ford, showing all the signs of its advancing years, frequently required emergency care. Preventive care was not, in my friend's opinion, either necessary or advisable. If his car wheels continued to turn in the right direction with reasonable certainty, that was all that was required.

When emergency treatment *was* required, Jack Sparrow took his conveyance to the service station in Okotoks. His visits were sometimes made during the evening hours. For the convenience of patrons, the owner of the service station had installed a light on top of a metal pole about six feet high, just outside the garage towards the main road. The garage owner was justly proud of this innovative customer service, its pole embedded in the ground at a spot compatible with the average driver's ability to back and turn a car.

Unfortunately, Mr. Sparrow was not an average driver. Usually when he arrived for emergency care his car barely crawled into the service bay; but, an hour or so later, with the engine functioning once again, it would be backed out with the speed of a thunderbolt, and since the brakes were never too reliable, the service light was quite regularly knocked over, and not infrequently, smashed.

Over the months the frequency of this mishap began to prey on the garage owner's mind. Retribution, rather than restitution, began to occupy his thoughts. His opportunity came one winter evening when Jack made one of his emergency visits.

The car was attended to. It was then backed out by its owner with its usual celerity, and as usual it knocked over the emergency light. Jack Sparrow, always the gentleman, returned to the garage to make his apologies for this quite unforeseen accident.

"Just keep him talking for a bit," whispered the garage owner to Walter Malinski, the mechanic. "I've got a bit of work to do outside."

Pleasantries concluded, Jack re-entered his car and drove off. With him went the pole and its light, suspended, like a beacon on a bad night, feet above the car.

"What the . . . ," exclaimed Walter.

"Best piece of welding I've ever done," said his boss. "And the fastest. While you were talking to him I welded the pole to his bumper. I bet you he doesn't notice it tonight – but, boy, I'd give a lot to be there tomorrow morning when he does! It's a present to old Sparrow," he added. "He's knocked that goddam light over so often, I thought he might as well have it as a souvenir!"

A couple of weeks after Mr. Sparrow had anesthetized himself for his tooth extraction, I was sitting in our front room, waiting for patients to arrive. None did, during our advertised office hours, and I was about to suggest to Janet that we go for a walk, when I heard a car coming along Elma Street. It was some distance away at first, but even then I could hear, quite plainly, that this car was hardly in good operating condition. The engine was running loudly but irregularly and there was a scraping noise that grew louder as the car drew nearer. This noise I diagnosed, and later confirmed, as being produced by the exhaust pipe trailing on the ground. There was, I might add, a town by-law against exhaust pipes that trailed on the gravel. But Jack Sparrow's exhaust trailed its way along, month in and month out, unchallenged.

Suddenly, as the noise reached a crescendo that suggested the car was level with our house, there was silence, apart from a few whimpers and shudders as if the engine were protesting this cessation of activity. Shortly afterwards there was a knock at our front door, answered by Janet. Very quickly she returned and said,

"It's Mr. Sparrow. He wouldn't come in. He's waiting for you in his car – says he wants to take you for a run."

When I reached the sidewalk my ex-dental patient was sitting behind the wheel. He reached over and opened the passenger door.

"Get in."

Before accepting this kind invitation I noted that the back seat contained a gasoline can, a selection of ropes of various thicknesses, a blanket or two, a spade and two immaculate, high-powered rifles.

"Where are we going?"

"I'll show you."

"How long will we be?"

"About four hours, give or take a bit."

"I'd like to tell Janet."

"If you have to."

Having given Mr. Sparrow's explicit information to my better half, I rejoined him. The engine rumbled and coughed into life and we drove down Elm Street, the cacophony of rumbling engine and scraping gravel making us the cynosure of all eyes. He jerked his head towards the back seat.

"I suppose you know how to use one of those things?"

"A rifle? Oh yes."

"Good. We'll soon see how good you are."

"What exactly are we going to do?"

"We're going hunting. You need a bit of meat to put on the table and I wouldn't mind some myself."

"That's very interesting. You don't need a licence to hunt in Canada?"

"I don't need a licence."

"Oh! Where do you hunt as a rule?"

"Any goddam place I feel like hunting."

"And where today?"

"We're going to the E.P. Ranch."

"The *E.P. Ranch*?" I repeated. "That's famous, of course, even in England. That's the Edward, Prince of Wales Ranch? Very interesting!"

"Right. And I happen to know where there's a nice herd of elk with a few more bucks than they need. And I happen to know," went on my new friend, "that the game warden is out of the area, at a convention in Banff, and so's the corporal of Mounties – and those young cubs of his are running up and down the highway handing out speeding tickets when they'd be better employed enforcing laws that ought to be enforced."

"Mr. Sparrow," I cried, "isn't there a legal hunting season in Canada, and isn't this all dreadfully illegal?"

113

"Dreadfully illegal?" he repeated, mincing his words a little unfairly, I thought. "It's as illegal as hell."

"But we might get caught!"

"You should always adopt a positive attitude toward life, young fellow," said the philosopher severely. "I've got no intention of being caught."

By now we had left Okotoks a mile or two behind us and were clattering our way into the foothills.

Suddenly the door on my side swung open, for no reason that I could think of.

"It always does that," said my companion. "Just bang it shut."

"Mr. Sparrow!" I cried in alarm. "If you get caught with a rifle in your hands, you will probably be fined – but if I get caught, I could be deported – isn't that true? I'm just a landed immigrant, a newcomer, I'm not even a Canadian. They could pack me back to England! And," I added, "the Prince of Wales Ranch of all places! My God!"

"That's the best damn place I can think of to hunt," said my guide. "And just because it belongs to the Royal family – that makes it all the better. Hell! The original owners of this land didn't hand out licences to their people. If an Indian needed meat on his table, he went and got a deer."

He eased the car into the side of the road and stopped.

"You're right," he said. "You could land in trouble. Mind you," he added, "there's not a cat's chance in hell that we'd be caught. Still – it's not worth the risk. I'll take you home."

Without another word, he turned the car in the middle of the road to the accompaniment of screeching brakes from an approaching vehicle. Mr. Sparrow eyed the driver admonitorily.

"You'd wonder where they learned to drive," he remarked to me, adding, "watch your door there. That wire isn't on right."

He drove me home, and as I got out at our front door, he said, "That was just too bad. We could have had a good afternoon out there," and drove off again with a parting nod.

Jack Sparrow, my friend for years to come, would have made an ideal buccaneer. Or as Molly, his wife, put it more gently – when she once said to me in that soft Scottish voice of hers, "I'm afraid, Morris, Jack was aye a bit of a non-conformist."

114

Chapter
Nineteen

When we first went to Okotoks there was no resident vet between the town of High River, fifteen miles to the south of us, and Calgary, twenty-five miles north. There was a lot of territory in between, and sometimes complications did arise and I would be asked to give emergency advice – but seldom by my ranching and farming friends. They, with one or two notable exceptions, treated my veterinary skills with great jocularity.

They would let me take care of their families, deliver their babies, but when it came to an expensive horse or cow, they had no intention of letting their family physician within even talking distance of the patient. They were wise men.

My veterinary practice – and a most unremunerative one it was – was limited to what is known in professional circles as "small animal work." It was usually carried on after hours, and it was all emergency work – often small dogs that had been run over by passing cars. At one time I had two dogs hopping around the town with one or other of their legs in casts. Besides being unremunerative work, it was also exasperating. My patients usually chewed their casts into a thousand pieces. Still, it was an interesting sidelight to country practice in the foothills of the Rockies, and my opinion with regard to animal husbandry was not always dismissed with cheerful derision.

It was early morning. It was also springtime in the Rockies just forty miles away, when the telephone at my bedside set up a steady clangor. It was five a.m. according to my watch, an unearthly hour to be roused, but no one had told that to the birds. There they were, dozens of them, on the bushes outside our bedroom window, chirping away like lunatics.

Levering myself onto my elbow and looking out of the window, I took grumpy note of the distant mountains. Bathed in the post dawn pinks and reds reflected from the rising sun, they were visions of beauty and magnificence. I was not in a mood to appreciate them.

"Gibson here."

"Doc, did I get you up? You sound as if you'd just wakened."

It was Jesse Hartland. I recognized his voice as soon as he spoke. He had a ranch a few miles outside town.

"It's five a.m., Jesse."

"So it is. Say, the morning's half over; listen – I need your help. It's urgent."

In an instant I was wide awake, my mind in a state of quick receptiveness.

"You know my brown gelding, doc? Well, it's foundered. I can't do a thing with it. It's just lying on the ground puffing and panting like a grampus. I can't get it on its feet at all. What should I do?"

"Do? Get a vet, Jesse, that's what to *do!*"

In hurt, almost aggrieved tones, my friend appealed to my better instincts.

"Come on, doc. You've got t'know something to do. And I can't get the vet. He's been out all night on a case. I've left a message for him. Just gimme your advice. That's all I ask."

There you are! How could I ignore such an appeal? Here was the one man – well, not quite the only one – but one man who valued my advice on veterinary matters, and I was on the point of rejecting his plea for help? I pondered the matter.

It has been my experience that when some of the locals talked of "foundered horses" the description covered a wide panorama of possibilities. Some of the earlier settlers had been retired naval officers. Perhaps they thought in naval terms, of ships, and their offspring were still confused.

A foundered horse, according to the dictionary, is one "suffering from laminitis, inflammation of a tender area of the hoof". For some reason that still defeats me, it can also be associated with overeating. The connection between these two very distantly related problems is a matter for conjecture – but not at the unearthly hour of five o'clock in the morning. The most dangerous possibility was some acute infection. Obviously fast action was needed.

"Do you have any penicillin out there?"

"I always have some handy."

"OK. Have you any brandy or whisky?"

"You know I have."

116

"All right. It could be an acute infection, so we'll take no chances and give it a shot of penicillin."

"Fine. How much?"

"This isn't my line, you know, but while you're waiting, why don't you give ten million units – into muscle."

"As good as done. What next?"

Suddenly I was aware of a tousled red head rising from the pillow beside me, and a hand shaking my shoulder and two utterly alarmed blue eyes looking into mine.

"Ten million units of penicillin? Have you gone mad? You'll kill somebody!"

I raised my hand imperiously, quelling – for the moment – my interrupter.

"Now, Jesse, whisky. A full cupful in a quart of hot water, plus about four tablespoonsful of sugar. Pour the lot down its throat." (We'd call that a hot toddy in Scotland – very efficacious for "owt that ails you" – as we'd say in Yorkshire!)

Janet was out of bed and reaching for her dressing gown. Jesse had gone to carry out my instructions. The telephone was replaced.

"Hold it! Hold it!" I told my alarmed wife. "It's a horse. I'm treating a foundered horse."

Alarm was swiftly replaced by indignation.

"A horse! And what do you know about horses? Have you gone out of your mind?"

"Darling," I replied, "this horse is down and out. The vet's been away all night. Jesse thinks it's had it. Now desperate illnesses require desperate remedies. Either this animal has some acute infection, in which case the penicillin might help, or else it's been into the oats and it's got some kind of bloat, in which case a good old Scotch toddy is going to give that gelding the most monumental burp of its life. Go to sleep, Janet. There's no more to be done."

And so, swearing at the cheerful, chirping cacophony from the bushes at the window, I drifted into sweet, dreamless sleep.

Then the phone rang.

"Yes," I snarled. "It's the doctor."

"I know that, doc," said the cheerful voice from the north side of the Sheep River, "and you're a walking wonder. It must

117

have been that penicillin. It's a miracle drug all right. He's up and about as bright as you please. So you can go back to sleep now."

Sleep? Grumpily I made a potful of tea. Still, I became philosophical. Of course it wasn't the penicillin that did it. It was a much older drug – the barley brew. A series of immense burps in all directions had saved the day, so I was told later.

My skill as a vet had been recognized at last. I had gained not just the gratitude, but the respect of a friend.

I did not know it then but my greatest case was, in terms of time, just around the corner.

"It's Mrs. Foggarty to see you," said Monica, adding enigmatically, "she says she can wait, it's not a medical matter."

The afternoon's work was underway. It was cold outside, well below zero, but the little waiting room with its colored settees and bright curtains, was warm and comfortable. And it was nearly full. A pile of snowboots lay behind the door and the clothes rack was engulfed by parkas. Cheerful records were being played on our gramophone, and soothed by the lilt of a Strauss waltz, tongues had loosened. There was a subdued but steady buzz of conversation as folks in from the country "visited" with one another.

The Foggartys were newcomers. They were city people, but Mike's ambition was to be a farmer. They owned a small acreage complete with house and outbuildings, and with those, a herd of Holstein cattle. Mike, a salesman, spent much of his time away from home and the farm was merely a weekend haven for him. I wouldn't have said it was any rest home for his wife. The children and the cattle kept her hard at work. She was a little wisp of a creature and I often wondered how she managed to cope with all her chores.

Mike, like many another city dweller, harbored the illusion that the countryman, surrounded by the beauties of nature, lives an idyllic existence. Mrs. Foggarty's dreams, urged on by the reality of toil and the prairie winters, had long since vanished. They lived a few miles out of town. It would soon be dark, and deciding that the occupants of the waiting room were content to talk, I saw her at once.

She was standing, swaying gently to comfort the little one she held in the crook of her arm. An older child, clutching at her mother's coat for security, watched me shyly.

"It's this stuff, doctor. I can't put any of it together and I thought you might help me."

In her outstretched hand was a paper bag containing bits and pieces of several veterinary syringes, the metal parts rusty, the glass opaque and cracked.

"They're just like surgical ones, aren't they? Could you put one together for me?"

That was a task beyond my ability, or indeed any human skill. Not one part of one of those antiques fitted another.

"Why d'you want a veterinary syringe?" I asked.

"Well, I've got a sick cow. The vet can't come from Calgary till tomorrow, but he's sure it's pneumonia and I've to give an injection of penicillin today."

"You've given injections to cows before, I take it?" I queried.

"Oh no! Never. But I'm sure I could do it. If you'd just assemble a syringe . . ."

"Look, Mrs. Foggarty. I don't think you should be doing this alone out there. Now you go home. I'll go to the druggist's, get a new syringe and this evening *I'll* come out and give the cow its shot."

Gratefully she accepted my offer and thoughtfully I completed the afternoon's work. I'd never given a cow a shot either, and I began to recall my days in England as "a pig man", when my patients at the very sight of a syringe would gallop into the corner of a sty, climb squealing on to one another's backs, and all of a sudden become possessed of the most demonic vigor.

But then, I comforted myself, pigs are very perceptive, surprisingly intelligent, edgy animals. Milk cows, by their very nature, are gentle, placid creatures.

The day's work done, I visited the druggist. My friend and colleague greeted my request for a veterinary syringe with quite unseemly mirth. Who was the lucky patient, he wanted to know. My unamused explanation met with a swift response. Mirth changed to alarm and Al firmly replaced the syringe on the shelf. Had I ever, he demanded to know, given a cow an injection?

"No, but suitably equipped, there was no reason why . . ."

My friend wasn't listening to me. He was talking to someone on the telephone, and then he said, "It's Tom Smithers. He wants to talk to you."

Tom was a rancher, a good one, and as the druggist knew, rather a crony of mine.

"Doc – what's all this about you giving a cow a shot of penicillin?"

For the second time that day, I explained matters and that gravelly voice at the other end commented, "If you have to be a boy scout then I'll be one too. I'll give that injection and you watch. Pick me up in half an hour."

"Tom – there's no need . . ."

"Have you ever given a cow an injection? No? Ever had a broken leg? No? Well, you were going to accomplish two firsts tonight, believe me." And he rang off.

Apologetically, Al said he hoped I wasn't offended, but he was a country boy himself and . . . I wasn't offended. I was relieved, and to this day I'm grateful.

When Tom and I reached the Foggarty place, we went straight to the barn. We knew which animal to look for, and there it stood in its stall, flanks heaving, head swaying. Tom's expert eyes quickly assessed the situation.

"The vet's right, doc. Let's give it that shot."

The cow was a pathetic, very unmenacing sight as my friend approached it, talking quietly. Listlessly it looked at him for a moment, as quietly he stroked its hide.

"Stand back, doc – over there. Now watch."

Tom was a big man. He was patting the cow's hind quarter and then with astonishing speed for such a bulky fellow, the injection was given and he leapt back beside me. And not a fraction of a second too soon, for that great black and white leg shot out and back with terrific speed and power. With horror I looked at where I would have stood to give the shot. A broken leg would have been the least of my injuries. The force of that kick would have killed an inexperienced man.

Grinning, Tom Smithers watched my expression.

"Every man to his trade, doc, but don't, for your friends'
sake, be a boy scout again – not with Holsteins."

The drive home was a silent one. Tom sat beside me, contentedly puffing at his cigar, snug in his parka, stetson clamped
firmly on his forehead. I contemplated the catastrophe there
would have been, had I not been forestalled in my foolishness.
My embarrassed thanks were cheerfully brushed aside.

"Forget it. I'll catch you sometime when I need you."

And he did, too.

Chapter
Twenty

A few weeks passed before I heard from Tom, but one evening
when the phone rang, he was at the other end. He cut short
my cheerful greeting. Indeed, he sounded rather indignant, and
his opening remark quite took me aback.

"Doc, if you've a patient with a broken leg, would you shoot
him?"

"Eh?"

"If you've a patient with a . . ."

I had heard Tom the first time and I said so.

"What I want to know is – would you give up on one of your
patients with a broken leg?"

"No, of course not, Tommy. Don't be ridiculous."

"What'd you do?"

"Why – I'd set it, of course!"

"Sure you would. Any self-respecting doctor'd set a broken
leg. Isn't that a fact?"

"Tom, you're speaking in riddles. What on earth are you
talking about?"

"I'm serious. I've a patient here with a broken leg. I've been told to shoot him. I'm damned if I'll do it. That's why I'm ringing you."

"Have you been drinking?"

"Never more sober, doc. Just mad. You see, I've just had the vet out from Calgary. It's one of my young bulls. It's been limping for a day or two. The vet takes one look at it, says the hind leg's broken and tells me to shoot it. Then he leaves. Hardly spoke a word to me, the son of a gun. Mind you, I wasn't just buddy-buddy with him either. I sure told him what I thought of his ideas on treatment."

"Oh! I *am* sorry, Tom. That's pretty rough."

"You bet it's rough. Do you know how much these bulls are worth? And this one's just young too."

Tom was a successful rancher and proud of his livestock. I tried to soothe him. Understandably he was upset. Obviously he wanted to talk to someone, and who better than his family doctor? Counselling patients in times of emotional stress is part of our stock-in-trade, and I listened sympathetically.

"Too bad, Tommy. Sorry to hear this."

"Yeah! Well there's nothing doing. I'm not shooting it. I'm going to set that leg, that's what I'm going to do."

"Tom – the vet must have had reason . . ."

"Don't tell me anything about the vet," interrupted Tommy. "I'm going to set that leg."

"Well, of course Tom, it's your bull."

"Right. That's why I'm goin' to set that leg – and you're going to help me."

"WHAT?"

"That's right. You made a pretty good job of Joe Stupik's leg an' if you can do it for Joe, you can do it for my bull."

"Now, Tom," I cried in the most unprofessional manner, "I'm damned if I am. I'm not going within twenty feet of your bull. Furthermore" – moral indignation was added to my mounting apprehension and terror – "I don't know anything about fractured legs in cattle. You forget it. Do you think I'm daft?"

"No, I don't. It's my bull and I won't shoot it. The goddam vet could have set it if he wanted to. I told him that too. Come on, doc, you wouldn't let me down, would you?"

"Tom," I pleaded, "I don't know anything about cattle. Why not get a second opinion from another vet?"

"You fellows all stick together. D'you know what the opinion would be? Shoot the bugger – that's what 'e'd say. Remember how I helped you with the Foggarty cow? I said I'd catch you when I needed you. Well, this is the day."

"Tom – one kick from that brute and I'll have an instant change of sex. I'll not do it."

"Scared, eh?"

"Of course not! Certainly not!"

"Well, then, I thought you were my friend."

"I *am* your friend. And as your friend, I'm telling you I don't know anything about broken legs in cattle, and if you're not happy, get another vet."

"Ah – but you know about broken legs in people. You know how to use that plaster of Paris stuff they use for casts?"

"Of course I do."

"There you are, you see. All I'm asking for is your expert advice. I'm not even asking you to set the leg. I'll do that if you won't. What I want you to do is show me how to do it, and put on the cast. I'm going to show that vet he was wrong. Come on, doc – you owe me. Besides, you're my friend."

So, of course, after supper that night, armed with yards of plaster of Paris bandages, and fortified by a well-earned lecture from Janet on my capacity for quixotic, not to mention foolhardy, action, I presented myself at my friend's home.

It was a cheerful rancher who greeted me, remarking within the hearing of two grinning ranch hands,

"I didn't really mean that about you bein' scared. Honest. I just felt you needed a bit of a push in the right direction. C'mon doc, the patient's in here."

He led the way across the snow-covered yard, rutted and frozen as hard as steel, to a small, ill-lit barn. Inside we gathered silently around the injured animal. Its belly cradled in a huge canvas sling ingeniously fixed to the roof beams by a system of chains, all four hooves were just clear of the ground. The broken leg looked little different to the others, but, my friend assured me, the animal was walking with great difficulty. On a rough table nearby were laid bowls of water, wads of cotton wool, and now the plaster bandages I had brought with me.

"Doc, the boys'll rope the legs. It won't kick. By examining it, could you tell me if it's a bad break?"

It was all very new to me, and it was a challenge and willy-nilly I became involved. Certainly there was a fracture, I said, running my hand along the leg, but it didn't seem to be a bad one. It was in good alignment – a clean break.

"Thought so," grunted Tommy. "How'd you set it?"

"It doesn't seem to need any setting, as far as I can see."

"OK. Let's put it in a cast."

So we set to work. It was a bitterly cold night, and there was little heat in the barn, but the work generated its own warmth. We slipped and slithered on the duckboards, pulling on ropes and chains, the ranch hands holding the leg steady while it was encased in roll after roll of plaster set over stout splints that kept the fracture in alignment. Eventually it was done. The patient, surprisingly docile, had even at times turned its head to observe the proceedings.

"Now," said the bonesetter, "he's going to stay that way, in that sling, with that leg off the ground till he's better. How long'll that be, doc?"

"I really couldn't hazard a guess, Tom – two or three months."

So, intrigued and amused, I went about my work. Weeks later I saw my four-legged patient again. He was one of the most pampered creatures I've ever seen, groomed and fed with loving care by the Smithers kids, and I remarked that he seemed content to spend the rest of his days in that sling.

Then, winter melted away. The snow disappeared, uncovering the faded brown and yellow grass of the fall before; the sun warmed the fertile soil and miraculously it seemed, we woke one morning to a world of blue skies and green grass. Then it was summer, and one day I called in at the Smithers' place. Tom was pleased to see me, and with an arm round my shoulder, propelled me in the direction of the corral. Six young bulls, placidly munching their feed, stolidly eyed us.

"Which is it, doc? Bet you can't tell!"

It was true. I wandered around, looking at right rear legs, while my friend kept the animals moving.

"Wonderful, Tom. It's been a complete cure!"

"But," said Tom, "I had to talk you into it, didn't I?"

Then the summer's heat departed as swiftly as it had come and soon we were into winter. Another year went by. Christmas was almost upon us, and with it the cocktail party season, always welcomed after the long days and nights of harvesting.

So one night, Janet and I drove to an outlying ranch. It was a jolly gathering. The pre-dinner drinks were generous, for our host and hostess, like most of their kind, were convivial people. A fire burned brightly in the great stone fireplace. Friends greeted one another, glasses in hand, then went their separate ways, "circulating" as they put it. Later, however, the ladies gathered in the sitting room, while the men congregated in the kitchen, though a few of us stayed politely with the opposite sex. Since one of them had launched into a dissertation on the growing of African violets, and gusts of laughter were coming from the kitchen, I felt my presence would hardly be missed if I joined the men.

They were clustered around an individual who seemed to be the source of their amusement. Quietly, I attached myself to the fringe of his appreciative audience. I recognized him at once. He was a well-known veterinary surgeon, from Calgary. He had a voice that would have done credit to any sergeant major on parade. For a moment, however, there was a pause. He was draining the contents of his glass amidst the encouraging titters of his listeners. Thus fortified, he went on.

"There I was at the MacCallums' place, with this bull lying on the ground. Smithers had sold it to him. I recognized it the minute I saw it – same bull. No doubt about it, I tell you. And of course the minute it mounted that cow, the leg couldn't take the weight and it broke all over again. Any damn fool could have told him it would. I'd told him to shoot it. He told me to go to hell – said if I wouldn't set it, he knew just the man who would."

He paused momentarily to quaff the contents of a fresh glass, pressed upon him by an admirer. But the more titillating details of his story had been told, and the audience was quieter now.

"And let me tell you," he bellowed, "that leg had been set by a professional – and the minute I find the crook, I'll have him disbarred, if it's the last thing I do."

125

At that moment, I recalled how the growing of African violets was an ancient passion of mine – much safer than the practice of animal husbandry – and thoughtfully I rejoined the ladies.

Chapter
Twenty-one

The city dweller doesn't need to pay too much attention to the weather. The countryman's life is sometimes ruled by it. In the city there may be inconvenience because of bad weather but services such as transport to and from one's work are rarely stopped. A bad snowfall on the prairie can create havoc. Traffic is brought to a halt. Schools can be closed, usually in good time for school buses to take the children home. With good weather forecasting, country children seldom have to spend a night or two in the homes of friends in town, but it still happens. Even the police can be immobilized. One has to experience the full ferocity of a prairie blizzard to realize its dangers, especially for the inexperienced or the unwary.

More than once I have traveled out to emergencies behind the snow plow laboriously clearing a path for my car, and in the worst conditions I have sometimes phoned the Mounted Police barracks. In some cases, such as road accidents, they relied on me as much as I relied on them and I never had to plead for company. Constables were ready to come with me in bad weather and I always appreciated the company of those husky young Mounties.

We always tried to interpret portents in the sky – that immense vault of heaven that is the Alberta sky. Even in summer there were warnings. Sudden clouds could mean hail and the ruin of crops, but it was the winter skies that we scanned most anxiously, for dark clouds gathering over the mountains or coming from the north could mean snow and cold. And that meant trouble for travelers, ranchers, and livestock. Every year or two it seemed that people – even country folk – caught unprepared were found frozen in their cars, and occasionally a farmer has succumbed to the cold on his own land close to home.

It was during our very first winter, late one dark night, that a farmer telephoned me to say he was worried about their baby. For some reason he was alone in the house. The baby had a high fever and he didn't want to risk taking it out on the roads even in a heated car. He had heard I did house calls. Would I do one now . . .

I asked for directions. His farm was ten miles away.

"It's easy to get here, doc, if you follow the instructions. Go straight west of town for four miles. Turn north for one mile. West again for two miles, then . . ."

I was busy taking notes. I was confused.

"Repeat your directions," I asked.

He went over them again. I still wasn't sure of them.

"I know what to do, doc. I'll ring all the neighbors along the route and get them to put their yard lights on. Just follow the directions and look for the lights. They'll lead you right to my place and I'll put the truck out on the road at our gate with its lights on. Then you'll know where you are."

Nowadays houses on "acreages" are scattered over the countryside, and they all have "yard lights" that go on automatically at dusk, but there were no such conveniences in 1955. There could be quite a distance between farms and the lights guided me safely to my destination. I dealt with the emergency and set out for home – but how, I wondered, was I going to get there? There was no moon to light my way and it was early morning.

Apprehensively I started off. I needn't have worried. The lights were still on. People had waited for me to return. As I passed each farm on my way home the yard lights were switched off. The only sounds were the steady hum of the engine, the sighing of the wind and the soft crunch of the snow beneath the wheels, but I never felt alone. It was like passing lighthouses in the dark.

Perhaps that journey was a good apprenticeship for the one that followed. It was the day before Christmas of 1955.

Among our new friends were the Gants.

The Reverend Waverley Gant was then the Anglican vicar of Okotoks. Dorothy, his wife, had confessed to Janet that she was worried abour her husband undertaking the arduous task of driving to three or four scattered country churches that evening to hold Christmas Eve services. In that weather, she said, the driving would be enough for most people, let alone holding church services. Besides, the vicar's car was a small one with a canvas top, hardly the "right thing" for the "30 below" and snow that he would have to contend with.

Janet quietly suggested to me that I should volunteer my services as chauffeur for the occasion. I was glad to do that and since Waverley indicated that he would be glad to have my company we set off on this ecclesiastical circuit, first to the village of Hartell nearly thirty miles away where the congregation awaited his arrival. I have often enjoyed my visits to beautiful old village churches in England. This was different. The church was a white painted wooden structure, an unadorned rectangle of a place with a roof on it, standing cold and austere in the snow.

But the small congregation greeted their priest warmly and his Christmas message reflected that warmth. Then back to Black Diamond for another service, and on to Millarville.

The Anglican church at Millarville is the oldest in Southern Alberta. Built at the end of the last century and standing in its churchyard with the gravestones of the first settlers clustered round it, it is a picturesque log building.

The vicar had been able to relax between services, and since we were men of about the same age and shared common interests, the journey was not boring. The snowfall was increasing and the road was covered with several inches of the stuff as we approached Millarville. We were late. I had had to drive more slowly than anticipated in order to avoid skidding, and I felt that the waiting congregation might be growing restless.

In order to help my passenger, I decided to deposit him at the church door, and drove into the church yard. But not very far. The car simply settled into a snow drift.

"Oh dear!" said Waverley. "I think you've done it this time!"

"Padre," I reassured him, "just you get into that service and leave me to the car. I'll back it onto the road."

From the church came the joyful sounds of Christmas carols lustily sung by, I judged, a pretty fair-sized congregation.

The vicar hurried off to his duties, and cheerfully I set about digging the snow from under the car wheels. That task completed, I backed the car toward the road. It went back easily – for about three feet, then settled into snow that was deeper than ever.

Out I got again with my shovel and repeated the process. This time, when I started the engine, the car slid sideways. I put my foot on the accelerator and put the gears into reverse. The wheels began to spin.

The congregation was quiet now and I got out to inspect the situation. The car was hub deep in snow. For an instant I forgot my whereabouts and audibly called on the Deity, but not in exactly the kind of tones the vicar would use.

There was an almost miraculous response. A voice said gently, "Can I help you, doctor?"

I looked over my shoulder. In my hectic efforts to free the car from the snow I had failed to realize that all was silence in the church. No wonder. Most of the males of the congregation, in parkas and fur caps, led by my friend the vicar had silently left the church and gathered round my car. My address to the Deity had been answered promptly, if rather embarrassingly.

"Sorry about that, vicar," I mumbled, abashed. "I didn't really mean to take the Lord's name in vain – especially in your own church yard."

"I'm sure He'll forgive you," Mr. Gant cheerfully assured me. "After all, you've done His work tonight. Come on, men, let's get the doctor's car onto the road!"

Suddenly there was a good deal of digging, much pushing and shoving and within minutes the old Chevvy was standing in the roadway and I was invited to join the congregation. If I wasn't given the place of honor, I was given something better – the best seat in the house, right beside the wood stove.

We were an hour late in getting to Okotoks and the midnight service. Not that anybody seemed to notice. The church rafters were resounding with the congregation's singing as we drove up to the church door.

"You don't need to attend this one," said my passenger, thanking me for my help and smiling, "you've got a credit account on church services at the moment."

"Merry Christmas to you and yours."

Chapter
Twenty-two

Education concerns every caring parent and Janet and I had given Catriona's Canadian schooling much thought.

Although there was a high school in Okotoks that served the town and surrounding district, it was small. Catriona had already shown signs of being a bright little girl. Were local standards of education adequate, we wondered? Should we be thinking of boarding school? Emigrants, especially Britishers, who tend to think their own educational system is second to none, often have this fear.

Our worries were groundless. Catriona's teachers were professional, very approachable and interested, and we speedily gained confidence in their ability to assess our daughter's attainments and guide her future education.

That June of 1955, shortly after we arrived in Okotoks, Miss Helen McKay invited the little one to attend school for the remaining weeks of the school term. Her class was composed of youngsters of her own age and Catriona said some of them were very bright – "especially the girls."

Anxiously we awaited further comments. Our daughter had never attended a coeducational school and in Okotoks, many of the boys showed little interest in the academic side of life. They regarded school as a waste of time, and said so in language that would have curled a lumberjack's hair.

Bewildered and alarmed at first by this awesome freedom of expression on the part of her classmates, Catriona soon began to view the situation with amusement. The boys were merely "showing off", going through an awkward period in their own lives and they meant no harm. Most of them were fine youngsters, proud of their western heritage with its emphasis on endurance and physical strength.

By the time they were teenagers many of them were skilled horsemen and could handle cattle and farm machinery expertly. After school the farm boys had chores to do, for the "hired hands" were rapidly disappearing, lured to the city by higher wages. Farmers and ranchers needed all the help they could get and as a rule their sons would rather be working in the fields than in the classroom. Some of these teenagers could build a house, install electrical fittings, drive tractors and take the engines apart if they had to.

It was a difficult world for us, and especially so for Catriona who had to spend her days at school among strangers, but we were quickly reassured by the way in which she adapted to her new surroundings.

There were very few private schools in Western Canada. The Canadian school system to some extent resembles that of the Scotland of my boyhood, when most children attended day schools managed by local authorities. We youngsters were, as they say in Scotland, "all Jock Tamson's bairns", where the lawyer's and the doctor's children sat beside the laborer's children. There was an admirable egalitarianism with an equality of opportunity for most.

In Scottish cities there were fee-paying day schools, but the English boarding school system was almost unknown. A bright child could receive a sound education at public expense up to university level. The not-so-bright, the late developers and those unfortunates who were forced to work to help support their families did not receive such consideration. They could leave school at fourteen and find employment. In its way it was an elitist system despite the egalitarianism, but it had been tempered by the realities of a hard world.

The one-room schoolhouse had been a North American tradition. The memory of them remained in Alberta in 1955. People would show old photographs of lonely huts standing on the bald prairie. There was usually a group of children, some of them on horseback, clustered round the doorway, in which stood the teacher, a girl not much older than some of her students. We knew several women who had started their careers as teachers in one-room rural schools. It must have been a gruelling job and yet I never heard a grumble from any of them despite their memories of blistering heat in summer with clouds of pestering mosquitoes, followed by the bitter cold of winter. Those young ladies taught children from toddlers to teenagers and all in the one room of the country schoolhouse. No wonder some of our patients would look around our transformed "Skye Glen schoolhouse" and say,

"To think that this is where I was educated!"

But the small rural schools, for all the wonders they had accomplished in pioneering times, were gradually disappearing. School districts were being consolidated, the children taken by school buses from their country homes to centralized schools in neighboring towns where there were better facilities for educational programs.

When we arrived, this process was still continuing, though many parents had received their early education in the old "one-room schools". The new system led to my being part of an interesting medical experience.

I had remembered one of our professors giving a lecture on how usually benign germs can become killers.

"They become killers," he said, "when they invade virgin territory."

He had been commenting on the deaths of a number of young Glasgow policemen from the complications of measles. The Glasgow Police Force attracted many lads from the isolated areas of the Highlands. Seldom exposed to this disease, these men had not acquired immunity to it. So measles, not usually a serious disease in childhood, became a deadly infection to these young men.

In Okotoks, the epidemic didn't kill anyone, but I saw some desperately ill men. They got mumps. There hadn't been an epidemic of this disease locally for several years. Mumps, a viral infection, is usually a fairly benign childhood ailment. While the children recovered quickly, some of their fathers developed very severe complications.

I'm still convinced that spending their childhood in the isolation

132

of the sparsely populated prairie, attending the one-room schools, and seldom being exposed to disease, these men had not acquired immunity to it.

I've often said that the bacteria and viruses have joined the jet set today. Germs need only board planes with their human hosts to be transported to virgin territory in some faraway country. But my patients in Okotoks didn't get their mumps from anything as exotic as a transcontinental jet. The virus came home on the school bus.

There were other educational differences to overcome. Rural schools were utilitarian institutions in the fifties. Very few of them had anything resembling a "school spirit". There were few physical training programs. The idea of spending money on playing fields or tennis courts would have caused many school board trustees to have apoplexy. They weren't parsimonious men. But they remembered the Depression, when teachers would work for little more than room and board, and local taxpayers had to struggle to survive, and they were haunted by the fear that it might all happen again.

Frugality had shadowed the lives of a whole generation. Changes would come with Alberta's growing affluence; there would be sports days and football fields and a broader outlook on education, but until that happened, not a penny was to be "idly" spent on such luxuries as gymnastic equipment or fancy laboratories.

And yet, the Okotoks High School, like many of its rural counterparts, has done well by its students. Former pupils have become successful farmers, engineers, officers in the Canadian Forces, physicians, lawyers and business executives – not a bad record for a prairie high school!

However, in that first year we had to think about our daughter and her ability to cope with the changes that confronted her. Once again we needn't have worried. She made friends quickly and although the team spirit of Tranby was far behind her and there were no field hockey games in Okotoks, Catriona had other challenges to face.

Mary Rowan and she soon became very close friends and after school there was a horse to be groomed. That in itself was an absorbing interest for both youngsters. Then there was the question of Canadianization. This didn't stop at the donning of blue jeans the moment school was over. Catriona began to acquire a Canadian accent. That was a painful business, more so for her parents than for young Gibson, as we listened to her agonizing attempts to speak like her classmates.

She had taken ballet lessons in England. She was a graceful little dancer too, but ballet was hardly all the rage in Okotoks. Instead she put Blackie through "figures of eight" on our front lawn. The front lawn wasn't the large expanse of beautiful green turf that we'd had in West Ella. It was just a large patch of prairie, baked and browned by the summer sun, but it served an admirable purpose, becoming an excellent horse ring.

And speedily we began to realize that our little British schoolgirl was showing signs of becoming a Canadian cowgirl!

Chapter
Twenty-three

Harry Lauder had a song that extolled the virtues of lying abed in the morning. Its words, sung in music halls all over the world, helped make him famous. Their sentiments have always appealed to me, and I have many a time been appealed to, to get out of bed in the morning early, without much result, unless presented with some emergency.

Perhaps it's a case of physiological need for sleep and rest. That has always been my argument when faced with the entreaties and then the commands of my wife. I do not face the mornings well, although for years I had to be in the operating room before 8.00 a.m., on several days of each week. I have never, however, taken umbrage when men I have thought to be my friends have referred, in my presence, to "the late Doctor Gibson".

And for some unearthly reason, when I am early for an appointment, trouble awaits me. So it was, one cold December morning, when I arrived at the hospital, prepared to do the "rounds" of the two patients then under my care. Between my car and the hospital door the ground had been covered in fresh overnight snow. I had reached the door and was shaking the stuff from my snowboots when Matron arrived.

"Just leave your boots on," she commanded, "and don't take your coat off. You're going straight out again."

"Oh? Where to?"

"You're just the guy we need," she said, showing an enthusiasm for my assistance that was novel to me.

"I am?"

"Yes. We've just had a message from Flat Top Mountain. There's been an accident on the oil rig there. They need doctors – and as fast as they can get them."

"Where's Flat Top Mountain?"

"West of High River. Forty – fifty miles. We're just packing Dr. Herring's car with plasma and every piece of equipment you're likely to need."

"What kind of accident?" I asked.

"We don't know," said Matron. "The radio connection was terrible. They just asked us to send doctors. It could be a fire, so as soon as Dr. Herring drives round that corner, the pair of you are on your way."

"But whereabouts *is* this oil rig on Flat Top Mountain, and is there a decent road in?" I asked.

"Oh, yes, there's a decent road in all right and then there's another road up," replied Matron, patiently.

"Up?"

"Yes, don't you know? The oil rig is right on top of the mountain."

"How far up is the top?"

"I'm not sure. Five – six thousand feet."

"My God. I can just imagine what kind of a road it is, too!"

"Not a bad idea to appeal to Him," agreed Matron, cheerfully, lifting her eyes as if in supplication. "You'll be all right. They drive trucks up that road every day. Here comes Dr. Herring. On your way, doctor. I'll phone your wife."

Dr. Friend Herring lived up to his name, and we were good

135

friends. He qualified in Medicine after World War II. During the war, as a young fellow, he had served as a petty officer, Royal Canadian Navy, on the North Atlantic. That experience inevitably adds a certain forcefulness to one's attitude to life. His car drew up beside me.

"Get in," was my colleague's greeting.

"Now, Friend," I said, at my diplomatic best, "this trip sounds as if it might be a bit rough, and that's a lovely new car you've got there. It's a shame to risk getting it dented. So why don't we take *my* car, and *I'll* do the driving, and you won't need to bother about your car. It doesn't matter about my car."

"You're damn right about your car," replied the good doctor, "That jalopy of yours wouldn't get us half way up. So we'll just use *my* car and *I'll* do the driving." Opening the passenger door a little wider, he said in the kind of voice that had roared commands above North Atlantic gales, "Get in."

We set off. Our scanty information was that there were severe injuries. Nowadays a helicopter might have accomplished in hours what took us until dark that night.

"The Mounties will be on our heels," my friend told me, "and the ambulance is going to meet us at the edge of town."

"What's the road like?" I asked.

"In summer it's pretty good," was the reply, "but I don't know about winter. It's a company road, so it's no highway!"

"What if something comes down when we're going up?"

"There are places where you can pull in," replied Dr. Herring. "But this morning we mustn't stop. If we do, we'll never get moving again. Besides, they know we're on our way. There won't be any traffic coming the other way. And we've got spades and chains."

Soon Friend pointed out Plateau Mountain to me. Amongst the neighboring peaks it was strangely level, and I could understand how it had become known as "Old Flat Top."

The ambulance was waiting at a crossroads; we waved to the crew as we sped past and they followed us a hundred yards or so behind.

"Friend," I asked, puzzled, "what on earth is an oil rig doing on top of a mountain?"

"I suppose because the geologists think there's oil underneath it," replied my colleague. "Oil's found in the queerest places."

The miles were slipping by. We were making good speed but the road was tricky. There had been snow overnight and the nearer we got to the mountains, the more there was. Underneath the snow there was ice, and the last thing we could afford to do was slip into a ditch, so my companion was concentrating on his driving, while I checked the equipment and supplies.

We had morphine. There was a selection of splints, slings, bandages, and bottles of plasma. We had been well supplied.

We speculated on what might lie ahead. Oil rigs can be dangerous places and in the years to come I would be called to more than one calamitous accident. Chains and hawsers can break suddenly under tension, flailing about with tremendous speed, devastating whatever lies in their path, while fires are a hazard and men can have limbs caught in machinery. An oil rig is no place for the weak-spirited and when accidents are reported to doctors, they are usually bad ones, for rig workers take pride in their toughness.

The flat grassland was behind us now. We were climbing, the spruce and pine trees all around us. The last few ranch gates came into view and then we were into the untouched forest, where the carpet of snow was thicker, the snow-laden spruce trees stood close together and the forest, dark and forbidding, began by the roadside.

"We'll be at the turn-off soon," said my companion, "and then it's on to the company road. That's when we'll really start climbing. But they keep the road clear the whole way up, so we should be all right."

I looked behind us. The ambulance was still in sight, plowing steadily along. Suddenly, there was the turn-off. In a few minutes we would be on the bare mountain and then I saw the ambulance skid, slew sideways and come to a stop.

"Friend," I exclaimed, "the ambulance has stopped."

"Too bad," grunted my colleague. "We can't stop for them. The police can only be a few miles behind. They'll stop and help them."

Steadily we forged ahead. The trees were thinning now. They had been a comfort to me, since they covered the steep slope to our right; had we skidded in that direction we would have been stopped. Friend's new car might have suffered but, I comforted myself, at our speed and with the trees so close, we wouldn't have gone very far.

Complacency, however, speedily turned to alarm. Abruptly we had climbed above the treeline. The road was steep, covered only with powdered snow and patches of ice, and there were no railings to prevent us going over the side. If it wasn't a precipice, the sight was enough to make my mouth go just a bit dry. One mistake, one skid and we would go rolling and tumbling down that steep slope into eternity.

Herring hardly gave the sight a glance. Slowly and carefully he guided the car up the track. Once or twice the rear wheels spun and my heart went into my mouth, but we reached the top. Coming out of the shelter of the mountainside, we made for the plateau.

There were low clouds all around us and peak after disembodied peak thrust through them, stretching as far as the eye could see. It was like looking down at a lost world, desolate yet beautiful.

We could see the oil rig and the buildings now, and I breathed a sigh of relief which suddenly changed to alarm as a tremendous gust of wind made the car swerve and rock. But we were away from the cliff side and despite the force of the wind we soon drew up at the main building. No sooner had we done so than men, roped together, ran towards the car, helped us out, thrust us inside this human chain and struggling against the wind, made for the door of the building.

The force of the wind took my breath away in those few yards, but once inside the hut, no time was wasted.

"This way, doctor," someone said to me. Friend went off to see another injury, while I followed the man who had spoken to me. Workmen, silent, grim-faced, standing in a group talking quietly, drinking coffee, watched us appraisingly as, emergency cases in hand, we strode down the corridor.

"There's nothing you can do, doctor," said my guide. "This man is beyond any help, but you'd better check him over."

My guide was right. There was nothing I or anyone could

have done. The corpse that lay on the bed was that of an older man, and I wondered if he was married.

"Yes. He's married," I was told. "Six kids, all at school. I just don't know how we're going to tell his wife."

I looked at the dead man's tranquil face, and thought, as I have done many times, of the strange ways of fate. Here, only a few hours before, had been a man, with thoughts and cares and pleasures. And now – nothing.

I turned away and went to see if I could help Friend. The group of men stood aside to let me pass. They had all been shaken by that morning's experience. There had been no fire, my guide told me, apologizing for the poor radio connection to High River.

"They were on their way up to work this morning. The truck skidded and went over the side. They all jumped, but two of them jumped too late."

"Where exactly did it happen?"

"You passed the spot on the way up. Maybe there were signs where it went over?"

"No," I replied grimly, "but I saw enough to scare *me*."

"Yeah. It's tricky all right. I guess the truck just started to slide and that was it."

Friend had been busy. His patient, shocked and in pain, had suffered a broken thigh. My help wasn't needed, and I stood talking to some of the men. I commented on the tremendous force of the wind. The rig workers nodded, and one said,

"These buildings are chained and roped to the ground. Maybe you noticed when you got here? Chains over the roof and staked into the rock. That's why we went out for you two men with the rope. If that wind had caught you it would have just blown you away. And there's a precipice where you'd have gone over," he added.

"As bad as that?" I commented.

"Only a few weeks ago, we had a hut built," he went on. "A good solid, heavy structure. It was dark when the work was done, so we left it till morning; we'd have chained it down then. It wasn't windy, but the wind came up later, and in the morning the hut had vanished. The wind just blew it right across the plateau and over the edge. It wasn't just smashed. Every plank was blown away."

The Mounted Police and the ambulance had arrived. After arranging for the transportation of the injured man to hospital, there was nothing left for us to do. It was afternoon, already dusk, and while neither of us relished the prospect of driving down that road in the dark, we were anxious to be on our way.

It was dark when we reached the shelter of the trees. The night sky was clear, a deep purple-blue and the stars glowed and twinkled far above. As we reached the flat grassland, I looked back. Far behind us the mountains were bathed in light, their crags and canyons soft in the shadows. It was a scene of tranquil beauty. But we had seen the cruel face of that beauty and would never forget it.

Years later, I recalled this adventure to a friend who said, "But think of all the money you must have been paid for that day's work."

Not so. The oil company disclaimed all responsibility for our modest fee. The accident had happened, not at work, but on the way to work, they said, so we should send our accounts to the patients.

I couldn't "bill" a widow. Dr. Herring's patient had accident insurance but left the hospital, giving no forwarding address.

So if Sir Harry Lauder, of whom we spoke at the beginning of this chapter, sang for *his* money, so did we, but to a different tune.

Chapter
Twenty-four

In the spring of 1956 we took stock of our position. Did we want to spend another winter in Okotoks? Did we want to stay there at all, and make it our home? There were pros and cons to consider.

We had spent a tremendously interesting nine months, seeing a way of life in Canada that is denied to many city dwellers, and I've often said we were privileged to experience this. We had found the frontier spirit that Dr. Christensen had spoken about, just as he said we would, and had responded to it. We had also seen real community spirit in action and were full of admiration for it.

"Neighbors" might live miles apart, but it was a case of "one for all and all for one" in times of trouble. In September of 1955 we had seen a farmer become so ill that he couldn't work. His crops lay in the fields, unharvested. But not for long. At a time when farmers work, not just from morning till night but sometimes throughout the night in order to get the grain in before the early snows, it was heartwarming to see how neighbors descended on that farm with their harvesting machinery. Half a dozen farmers and their wives, working together, had the fields harvested within days.

A house in town was badly damaged by fire. Neighbors contributed clothing and food, while others helped repair the damage.

Okotoks had a volunteer fire brigade – shopkeepers, mechanics and townsmen – who streamed in their cars or trucks to the firehall at the first wail of the siren, manned the fire truck and ran out the hoses like professionals. They were well trained and they had to be, for fire in towns where the houses are built of wood can be catastrophic, especially if there is a wind, when flames can leap from one building to another. We had seen a grain elevator almost explode and part of it go up like a bonfire before the Okotoks fire brigade brought the blaze under control.

Those nine months had been like a wonderful holiday in many ways – a total change from the daily grind of general practice in Hull. People weren't well off, but they were independent to a degree, and if they did not have ready cash for some small service, we would find a dozen or two eggs or a chicken brought to the door. Some people brought us little presents, butter and eggs, beef, just to introduce themselves and say they'd come to see us if we were needed.

There was a friendliness all around that was refreshing and enticing – but – we weren't making a living! We had earned just over $2,000 since arriving, and while living expenses were low, even by British standards, that kind of money would not keep the wolf from the door for long!

Indeed, the friendliness in itself was a problem. We weren't used to the easy assumption of first names in conversation, for instance.

"Mr. So and So," I'd still begin, when explaining some medical matter, to be corrected with, "my first name's Joe and that's the way it is out here."

And I was ruffled at first by the easy use of the ubiquitous "doc" until I realized it was the way of the countryman, and within months I would have had it no other way, not just accepting the greeting, but knowing that it signified a special kind of relationship I'd seldom known before.

Then there was the "western handshake". Those westerners shook hands with great frequency, we noted. In Britain, you didn't shake hands with an individual you'd seen a few days before. It simply wasn't done. But perhaps in the West the custom was a reminder of the days when neighbors lived miles apart and neighborliness was part of survival. We came to rather like it.

But Janet was at a disadvantage. She had been born and bred in a large city, and had always lived in cities. The smallness of Okotoks sometimes worried her, not from the point of view of isolation – though we knew several wives of immigrant doctors who could not stand the loneliness of prairie towns – but from the social side of life there.

She was that rare creature, a woman doctor and, as she said, a woman doctor in what was largely a man's world. There were few women doctors in Alberta then, especially in the country, and Janet had no intention of giving up practice.

"You see," she said, as we talked things over, "I have to wear about three hats. I have to be your wife, but it's also very important that I should be Catriona's mother. So I go to school and attend parent-teachers' meetings, and take an interest in school affairs, and in the little one's new friends. And when I do that, I'm Janet to people. Then when I work in the office, I'm a doctor. I have to be totally discreet about medical matters, yet if this is where we're going to live, I've got to strike a balance between my friendships as a mother of a little girl and as a physician in practice. In a close-knit community like this where there are few secrets, things aren't going to be easy!"

She missed her Hull University Women's Club, her literary society, and city life, with its anonymity and variety, but at the same time she was attracted to this new freedom. Life was stimulating in a different kind of way, she explained, for there was so much that had to be built out here. There was an excitement, a sense of optimism in this new land that gripped her.

Catriona had adapted very quickly to her new school, despite the initial "cultural shock" of being amongst boys for the first time. She had quickly made friends with several of the girls, especially with Mary Rowan to whom she was very close. And she was the proud possessor of a horse. She didn't really own "Blackie," who was on loan from the Indians. A neighbor had undertaken to find her a safe horse, and he had done an admirable job. "Blackie" either walked or stopped, but he was the right steed for our little one, who was happy, for "content can soothe, where'er by fortune placed."

But apart from our impecuniousness, we had another problem. We must find a house, or build one, before another winter. Our first home, so we were told, had originally been two small buildings, brought into town and joined together. There was nothing unusual in that. Once covered with stucco, the "two-part bungalow" looked attractive and had served us well in summer. But it was not insulated and became very cold in winter unless we stayed close to the stoves.

Catriona's little bedroom had a clothes closet in it, and that spring, we found the clothes nearest the outside wall encased in a film of ice where moisture had condensed, then frozen. We couldn't spend another winter there.

We had made friends in Calgary, and they asked us why we were both so adamant about remaining in Okotoks when we could either set up in practice in the city or join one of the clinics there, but our greatest predicament arose when we received a phone call from Saskatchewan. A senior partner in one of the province's quite prestigious clinics offered us both appointments in Regina, with a free, modern house "thrown in". He'd give us a couple of weeks to think it over, he said. It was a tempting offer. I told a friend about it. His reply was swift.

"I *came* here from Saskatchewan," he said, "and so did the half of Okotoks. The winters there are worse than they are here. Just stay where you are. Things'll work out."

I hoped they would. I didn't want to leave. I was learning something every day, and the work, even the winter weather, was a challenge.

Then, quite unexpectedly, we received word that $10,000 could be transferred from England to our bank in Canada. It was the beginning of a gradual change in our fortunes. Suddenly we felt wealthy, and we decided that we would build our house at once – but it must be built on land where we had a view of the mountains.

Chapter
Twenty-five

We had learned a lot about the West in that first year and had acquired an "extended family" before it was over.

First of all, my mother joined us in Okotoks, wisely insisting on having the independence of her own home. Our anxieties about her ability to cope with a new land were groundless, for she was immensely interested in meeting people and at seventy-six became an enthusiastic Canadian.

In that same year, as Catriona put it in her schoolgirl way, Mary Rowan "joined the team". It is strange how circumstances will bring people together.

Alberta can be a harsh and cruel country even during the most beautiful summers. Okotoks is in the "hail belt" and every summer, it seemed that just when the wheat was ready for harvest, there would be a hailstorm. The first ominous clouds would gather, grey and black against the calm blue sky, far to the west.

Then anxious eyes would follow them as the cumulus built up over the mountains, the first shafts of lightning, forked and dangerous, streaked towards the ground, and the rumbling of thunder disturbed the cattle. Instinctively they would bunch together, often dangerously close to the fence line. The horses, already apprehensive, would begin to trot about, tossing their manes and whinnying, while the hail clouds, nearer now, caught in the vortex around them, would begin to circle high above.

In the distance the first sheets of hail would begin to fall, like grey curtains draped from the skies. Harmless enough at that distance, they would fall on the forests. But soon the storm would be closer, the sky above black and foreboding, with the clouds circling and whirling like mad things. The first few drops of rain would fall, followed within seconds by the hail. In sheets, with hailstones as large as golf balls, it would destroy field upon field of crops, indiscriminately leaving a trail of devastated land behind it. Where moments before there had been golden grain, swaying gently in the breeze, there would be only smashed and dirty stubble.

The lightning could kill cattle, especially near barbed wire fences, while horses, tortured by the pelting hail, would gallop madly about, bucking. Windows would be broken, car roofs dented, flowers and shrubs destroyed, trees stripped of their leaves as the hail lashed the ground like a giant flail and all in a few minutes.

Farmers would be "hailed out" sometimes two or three years in a row. There was no organized crop insurance. Many farmers preferred to take their chances with the weather, and I never knew an unlucky farmer show self-pity. Grimly they would seek some kind of employment until the next spring, when they could return to their beloved land.

Mary Rowan, Catriona's little friend, lived on a farm about six miles west of Okotoks. Jim, her father, always said he'd been lucky as far as hail was concerned, but that summer their house was almost demolished by lightning during such a storm. The bolt hit the roof, blew a hole in it and blasted its way through what had been until that moment a comfortable, spotlessly kept family home, destroying everything in its path. The house was uninhabitable and the Rowans moved into a small cottage in Okotoks.

It was there that Mrs. Rowan showed the first signs of the illness that would lead to her death within a few months. Their daughter Mary, a slender, graceful child, was a few months older than Catriona, and already her close friend. As Mrs. Rowan's condition worsened, Mary spent more time with us. Their farm home had received almost irreparable damage, and though Jim, then a man in his sixties, felt he could continue to live there with his two sons, a little girl of twelve was another problem altogether.

The matter was solved when Janet, who was Mrs. Rowan's doctor, asked her if she would like Mary to live with us, where she could attend school more easily. Mrs. Rowan, deeply worried and knowing she had only days to live, gratefully accepted the suggestion.

And then, I had a commitment to keep. I had promised Catriona that she would have a pony of her own, and I began to look around for a replacement for old Blackie who had gone back to his Indian owners. A hundred dollars would buy a pretty good horse, and eventually I settled on a well broken, four-year-old gelding.

The girls promptly christened him "Peanuts", perhaps since that's what I paid for him! He was to be shared by all of us until I could afford to buy "Gray" a few months later. As it turned out, I never spent a hundred dollars more happily. Jack Sparrow forbade me to buy a saddle. He insisted that I accept his own cavalry saddle with riding boots to match.

Peanuts was a lovable, wily character and quite inseparable from the newest member of our little group. When we left Hull we'd had to find a home for Prince, our collie. It had been an emotional wrench and Janet and I decided there were to be no more dogs.

"It just followed us," said the girls in unison one day when I pointed accusingly at the bedraggled, miserable-looking creature at their heels. "We couldn't chase it away – honestly – it just kept coming after us. It's awfully hungry."

"Well, you can just lose it when you go back to school after lunch," I replied. "If I feed that stray once, it'll never leave!"

146

It never did, of course, and what a friend "Rough" proved to be! He was mostly collie, with a collie's intelligence and loyalty to match.

The little procession of Mary on Gray and Catriona on Peanuts seldom left our garden without Rough trotting alongside. Friends, I've heard it said, often develop similar likes. Rough developed a taste for Peanuts' oats, and they were often to be seen together, nose to nose at a handful of oats on the ground. One morning, with Peanuts tethered, I put a little heap of his favorite delicacy on the grass to keep him occupied awhile. No sooner had the horse started to nibble than Rough, who had been sitting a few feet away, decided he was not going to be excluded from this occasion. The pair of them seemed to be in competition to see who could eat the most oats in the fastest time.

Janet and I were watching from the kitchen window when quite deliberately Peanuts picked up his companion by the scruff of the neck and heaved him about six feet away. Then he stood and looked at the collie before returning to his nibbling.

On the other hand, Rough would sometimes take one of his friend's reins in his mouth and lead him to me.

In the years that followed I would often go riding on my own. I was spoiled – to this day I have difficulty saddling a horse – for one or other of the girls would "saddle up" for me, and off we'd go; Peanuts, myself and Rough. Sometimes I'd dismount, tie Peanuts' reins to the pommel, let him nibble at the grass, and stroll ahead, while Rough sat beside his pal. Not once in all those years did the horse desert me, and he never let me get too far away. I used to watch him with amusement, for periodically he'd stop cropping and look up to see where I was. Then he'd thunder along toward me at a gallop. It was unnerving at first to hear his hooves pounding on the ground, but he'd always slow down a few feet behind me, then nudge me in the back, sometimes none too gently.

Then it was time for me to remount.

The beautiful weather of that second summer seemed as if it would last forever. Then, in mid-September, there was a snow-fall that lasted a day and vanished; a few days later, a sudden frost. The mosquitoes were gone, flowers wilted, and the trees, almost overnight, became a blaze of color – golds and reds and yellows. But soon the leaves fell and the trees stood naked in the warm sun of the "Indian summer". The birds had gone, winging their way south, fleeing from the coming winter.

One afternoon in early November, I was asked if I would mind visiting a farm a few miles out of town. A Mr. Havercroft had a chest infection and was confined to bed. I was happy to travel a few miles to see the old gentleman, for I have always believed that it is important to treat some patients, especially the elderly, at home.

The afternoon sun was still warm, though its warmth had been fleeting of late, I had noticed. I had driven into the farm-yard, got out of the car and lifted my emergency case from the seat, when suddenly I shivered. The wind from the north had a chill to it, and I was wearing summer clothes.

My patient was soon attended to, and I left, glad to get into the shelter of the car. A few flakes of snow were drifting down from an almost cloudless sky, and I made a mental note to wear an overcoat that evening.

Two miles from home, I decided to call on one of my new friends who had often suggested that we have a beer together, and since Janet had told me she would have supper ready within the hour, I had good time to accept this invitation. Perhaps I enjoyed his hospitality for a little longer than I had intended, for when I emerged from the house I was astounded at what con-fronted me.

The ground was covered with snow, already piling up against bushes, fences and my car. The sky was almost black. The snow was no longer falling gently. In thick clouds, obliterating any sight of the driveway or the road a short distance away, snow streaked past, driven horizontally by that icy wind which con-stricted my forehead as if by a band of steel. I gasped for breath, my chest tight, as I struggled to the car.

I was only a mile or two from home, but that journey became a nightmare. The car was like a refrigerator. I couldn't see the road ahead. The roadside had vanished in a snowy fog, and I knew I dare not leave the car, and that the car must keep going.

But in the end, crawling along, hoping that the windshield wiper would keep working, I drew up at our door.

Janet was distraught. Like myself, she had never experienced an early fall blizzard.

"Where in God's name have you been?" she cried. "You should have been home an hour ago! Don't you know what you've done? Every man on the Gladys Ridge is out looking for you. When you didn't come home and that dreadful storm came up, I phoned the Havercrofts. They said the way you were dressed you wouldn't survive if your car got ditched or you got lost. All their neighbors are out searching the sideroads."

I had been taught a lesson and I never forgot it. From then on, I prepared for the winter long in advance. I kept proper clothing in the car, a sleeping bag, candles and matches – for a lighted candle will give out enough warmth to keep a man alive if his engine fails. And if I went any distance on a night call in bad weather I'd phone ahead and give the approximate time of arrival, repeating the ritual on the return trip.

Alberta winters are often as magnificent as the summers, posing no threat to people who are properly clad and aware of weather changes, for the sun shines almost continuously during the day, it seems, and prairie people love its brightness, even at forty below.

It is the unexpected blizzard that poses the danger. Three nurses returning to High River from a reception in Calgary were caught in such a sudden storm a few weeks after my adventure. They were lucky to escape with their lives.

The Mounted Police had no illusions about the weather, and did not hesitate to turn travelers back to town or forbid them to leave, if conditions deteriorated badly. But it all added a challenge to one immigrant's work!

149

Chapter
Twenty-six

We were also beginning to see more patients at this time. Young married women were inquiring if I would attend them when they had their babies. It was obvious that we were being accepted as members of the community.

When Jim MacDonald, of Okotoks' general store, heard of my ambition to build a house, he advised me to approach Mrs. Catherine Hogge, who lived on top of the hill and owned several building lots around her house.

"I don't think she'll sell one," said Jim, "but it's worth a try. She's quite the lady is Mrs. Hogge – very independent and not the kind of person you argue with. She's a widow, and her daughter-in-law, who's also a widow, lives with her."

After introducing myself by telephone, I went to interview this formidable lady. I found a tiny, Dresden-doll-like figure, with two of the bluest eyes I have ever seen. She was eighty and still a pretty woman. Sitting in state in her chair when I arrived, she invited me to sit opposite her while I explained my mission.

She listened without interrupting me, and when I had finished telling her how we wanted to stay in Okotoks, but only if we could build where there was a view of the mountains, she sat for a time, silently looking at me, until I began to feel uncomfortable.

Suddenly she smiled.

"I never could understand why everybody has to live down in that valley," she said, "when they could have this view. I suppose in the old days settlers thought that down there they'd get shelter from the winds. Come over to the window."

She rose and stood, looking out. There, below us, was the town, the trees and glimpses of the silver thread of the river, the Valley of the Sheep, and far to the west, the mountains.

"It's God's country you've come to," she declared. "I came here in 1883, you know. I was the first white girl in this part of the world – did you know that?"

"No!" I replied in astonishment. "But how did you come? And where did you come from?"

"My father, Morris Stewart, a Scotchman like yourself, came west from Quebec. We came by train to Winnipeg. That's where the railway ended. The rest of the way we came by Red River cart – a lot of it I rode on horseback." She smiled as she said, "You should have seen Winnipeg then – it was just a wee bit of a place, a thousand or two people – and half of them red-coat policemen."

"The Mounted Police, you mean?"

"That's right, the North West Mounted Police. And they were needed too."

"For fear of Indians?"

"No!" she laughed, "I was never afraid of Indians, even later when I was a young woman and they'd come to the door begging for food, poor folks, and I'd be alone. No," she went on, "but I was many a time afraid of whites."

"What was that journey like?" I inquired.

"It was eight hundred miles across the open prairie," said Mrs. Hogge, "and no roads. We drove the wagons through the grass. There were a lot of us in the wagon train, as the Americans called them, and we were half eaten by mosquitoes. We stopped at the Gladys Ridge just east of Okotoks in the winter of 1883 and we stayed there and homesteaded. But that first winter we lived in two tents – a small one inside a big one."

"It's a wonder you weren't ill!"

"It was healthy even if it was cold. But on the way out I lost a younger sister. We were coming across the prairie, with all the carts in a line and some of the men riding ahead, when we saw this big circle of Conestoga wagons ahead – covered wagons they're sometimes called. They were Americans of course, coming up from the south. A lot did that. There wasn't any sign of life and we wondered if they'd been attacked by Indians, so we all bunched up together – and then we saw three men ride out of the circle toward us. They stopped a ways off and shouted to us not to come near. They had some sickness and the children were dying. I rode up beside our men. The Americans said they were short of water and if we could leave them some they'd be grateful. I can see it still," she said. "That circle of wagons on the empty prairie and these men riding toward us. We didn't know what it meant. We just stood there, waiting.

"The women talked it over. They said they couldn't leave folks like that without help and some of them went over to see what could be done. Two or three days later we started getting it. That's when Milly died. A lot died. They were buried on the prairie. When it was over we went on again."

She smiled at me. "There weren't any doctors on the wagon trains, you know!"

I suppose the infection was diphtheria. Diphtheria epidemics, even in my student days, were dreaded. Children could be alive and bright one day, develop an insidious and deceptively mild sore throat the next and be dead within a few days. Such an experience on the trackless prairie, far from help or home, must have led to dreadful despair, and I looked at this slender, delicate little creature with growing respect and interest.

"Well, that's enough of that!" she said. "So you want to buy some of my land, eh?"

"Yes. I would like to, but perhaps you'd like to think about it?"

"I have thought about it," was the reply, "and I'll sell you the plot to the north of the house – on two conditions. You'll build a nice house and not a shack. And you won't plant many trees. I just don't much like trees," she explained. "They spoil the beauty of the wide open spaces."

That was one way to look at it, I thought. In Okotoks there seemed to be about three varieties of trees of any size, and how I longed at times to see an oak or an elm.

"Is that a deal?" said Mrs. Hogge.

"There's a question of money," I reminded her.

"Well, there's the land – name your price," was the reply. "I paid eight hundred dollars for all of it."

"Well," I said hesitantly, "would it be fair to offer you eight hundred dollars for the land you'll let me buy?"

"Done," said the lady, and thrust out her hand like a man.

"I'll have a lawyer draw up the necessary papers, Mrs. Hogge."

"I don't need a lawyer," was the immediate, emphatic reply. "There's no lawyer'll draw up any agreement that's better than the handshake of an honest man – you *are* an honest man, aren't you?" she continued, with that mischievous smile that Janet and I would get to know so well.

"Just give me your check and that's all we'll need. And if I were you, I'd start building as soon as I could. The season's short, you know, and you don't want to get caught out with an early winter."

She walked on to the lawn with me and looked across at the land she had just sold. Smiling, she said, "I know they say I'd never sell any of this – but I've sometimes thought it would be nice to have a neighbor. You'd better bring your wife and your little girl to meet me. I've a feeling we'll get on together."

Chapter
Twenty-seven

I speedily realized that Mrs. Hogge, for all her years, was a lady who knew exactly what she intended to do in most situations. She was a determined and, for all her apparent fragility, sometimes a formidable woman, but her firmness was offset by her wit and sense of humor.

The next time I went to see her about the lot,

"You'll need a garage," she told me, as we stood outside her house. "Now I have a chicken coop just behind the house, but I don't have any chickens. The coop would make a perfect garage, so I'm going to throw it in with the building lot. All you'll have to do is move it over to your place."

I thanked her for her kindness and pointing to the garage that stood beside her house, remarked that probably she just kept the gardening tools in it nowadays. After all, I thought, at eighty, she was hardly likely to need a car.

Mrs. Hogge appeared to have read my thoughts. Those china-blue eyes of hers looked straight at me. Pointedly she said,

"I keep my car in there."

Hurriedly I replied to the effect that I hadn't seen her driving around town and assumed . . .

"If you'd seen me driving around town," said Mrs. Hogge, "you wouldn't have forgotten. Would you like to see my car?"

Without waiting for a reply, she opened the garage doors. There, in shining splendor, stood her automobile. It was spotless. No doubt it had been the envy of her neighbors thirty years before. It was a black model A Ford with a canvas roof and large wheels that made the car stand so high off the ground, it seemed to me its owner would need a stepladder to get in – or out – of the thing.

I gaped at it.

"But," I cried, making a second blunder, "surely you don't *drive* this . . ."

"D'you want a bet?" asked the lady.

"Well, of course," I replied, "I realize that you must drive. It just seemed . . ." my voice trailed off.

Two very blue eyes watched me steadily.

"D'you want a bet," Mrs. Hogge said once again.

"What kind of a bet?" I asked cautiously, having realized by now that this old person was no lightweight in terms of will-power.

"I'll bet you," she went on, "ten dollars that I can drive this car right out of that garage this very minute. In fact, I'll take you downtown, pick up my groceries and drive you back. Will you take me on?"

Courtesy demanded that I accept.

"You wait here," commanded the gambler, "while I go into the house and put a hat on. I'll be right back."

Briskly she strode into her house, speedily re-emerged and indicated that I should take the passenger seat. She went to the front of the car.

"What are you going to do?" I asked.

"Well, I'll have to crank it, of course."

"But Mrs. Hogge," I cried in alarm, "you'll break your wrist or something!"

"Young man," replied my new friend, "I'll do nothing of the sort. This car is in perfect condition. And don't," she said emphatically, "offer to crank it for me. I couldn't take the responsibility. Just watch."

With great confidence she swung that antediluvian handle. Immediately the engine sprang into action.

"Perfect condition, you see," she said matter-of-factly. "Now we'll go downtown."

Effortlessly she backed the car out of the garage onto the grass track, turned it in a wide circle and then, in splendid state, high above any plebeian automobiles that passed us, we drove down the steep Okotoks hill and into town.

A spectator with a literary turn of mind might have remembered the poet's words:

> Like towering falcons aim
> At objects in an airy height,
> The little pleasure of the game
> Is from afar to view the flight.

Her errands quickly completed, Mrs. Hogge drove back up the hill, to my wonderment handling the old-fashioned gear lever with dextrous ease. With all the deftness of a veteran she drove the car into the garage and applied the brakes, leaving only inches between the front bumper and the wall.

Thrusting out her hand, she said sweetly, "That'll be ten dollars, doctor."

When I informed the town council that we would be building on Mrs. Hogge's land, they were enthusiastic. There hadn't been a house built in Okotoks for years but with a resident doctor in town, other folks might feel encouraged to build. However, there was one small snag. The council had joined the Calgary and District Planning Commission. They could not give me permission to build without seeking the Commission's approval, and suggested that I should go into Calgary for an interview, accompanied by one of their number who would officially support my application.

That seemed straightforward enough, and I set about finding a builder. We decided we should employ local people, and since

155

Mr. Jack Brown was highly recommended to us, we spoke to him.

Jack considered the proposal.

"Now, don't go away mad," he said in that quiet way of his, "but I've never built a house. I've built a lot of chicken coops and some barns. But never a house."

"Mr. Brown . . ." I began.

"Jack," said Mr. Brown, interrupting me. "If you start calling me Mr. Brown I'll get an inferiority complex and that's not good for a man. Now I think I could build you a house – if it's not too fancy."

"My wife has drawn up some plans of what she'd like," I told him. "There's nothing elaborate in the design. We'd like to build something that'd fit into the landscape – ranch style, looking west. Three bedrooms, a decent-sized living room and a kitchen. Something like that."

"Well," drawled our contractor, "I should be able to do that. There's not much difference between a house and a hen coop when all's said and done. But there's one big point – that wife of yours. Is she easy to work with?"

"Oh, very easy," I assured him.

"Not likely to get mad if the walls blow over, for instance?"

"Jack – are you having me on? I mean to say . . ."

"No, doc. I'm sure I can do it. With my experience in hen coops it should be easy. We should get started soon, though. I don't want to be working in the snow. You just tell me when you're ready and I'll be set to go. I'll select the lumber. You pay for it, and pay me my weekly wages. How's that?"

We shook hands on the deal. I arranged with Walter Thompson to dig out the basement with his bulldozer.

"You've got to have a basement out here," said Jack. "It's the basement that keeps the rest of the house warm. That's where you keep the furnace. And it's the cheapest room you'll ever build."

My next step was the matter of an interview with the planning commission. Jim Tucker was elected by his fellow councillors to accompany me.

"It'll just be a formality," said Jim. "They'll be delighted to

156

think that after all those years, Okotoks is getting a new house built, and getting a doctor of its own again."

In high spirits, Jim and I drove into Calgary and presented ourselves at the offices of the planning commission, where we were referred to the appropriate officials.

They were Britishers and it became obvious as I spoke to them that they had not been in Canada any length of time. They knew no more than I did about the vagaries of climate in the Western plains. My heart sank immediately. They obviously intended to take their duties very seriously, and after listening to our proposals, maps were produced and with grave nodding of heads and pursing of lips, we were informed that the project could not go forward. Permission to proceed, we were told, might be given after due process of deliberation.

I'd heard that kind of official jargon before and in the same accents, but diplomacy, I thought, might still prevail.

"How long will it take to come to a decision?" I asked.

"We don't know. Possibly a few months."

Jim explained that the council was anxious that I should build at once and I exclaimed,

"But if we have to wait for a few months it'll be winter! And my builder will leave me!"

"They all say that," was the rejoinder.

"How long," I asked, "have you two fellows been out here, anyway? Have you ever *experienced* a Canadian winter? Have you ever even *been* to Okotoks?"

No, they said, they didn't know much about Okotoks but they had "plans" for Okotoks and permission to proceed was denied. Implementation of their "plans" was to come nearly twenty years later!

Finally I announced that at 6.30 the following morning, Walter Thompson would start up his bulldozer and that if my bureaucrats presented themselves at the site with legal documents, I'd be pleased to peruse them.

The next morning dawned. I consulted my watch. It was just 6.30. Walter started his engine and I gave the word. The work began. It was mid-morning when an official-looking car drew up and a gentleman in a business suit alighted and walked toward me. I walked toward him.

157

"You're late," I snapped, "and if you don't have something to prove that you can stop me, then I suggest you get off my property."

He was quite taken aback and began to retreat to his car. Then he turned,

"Stop you?" he said in a puzzled way, "I'm not stopping anything, sir. I'm from the gas company. Mr. Brown phoned yester . . ."

"My dear fellow," I said, taking his arm, "*Do* please forgive me. I had forgotten about you. Of course you must put the gas line in."

Building that house was the best advertisement we could ever have had. People came from miles around to see it being built and to offer Jack advice, all of which that worthy listened to with great good humor.

If ever a house was built with loving care, it was that one. Because the building season lasted for only a few months, Jack was determined that his project would be finished before freeze-up. Janet handled the design. I handled the budget – with all the hilarity of a kirk elder counting the Sunday collection. And Jack showed an unexpected talent for diplomacy in his dealings between Janet's flair for design and my genius for frugality. True, that same genius once left the lady without stairs from her kitchen to the basement, and in the end we had to build a porch to accommodate the stairs we did build, but those were minor points.

When it was finished, the house was a warm and comfortable place. The living room, lined with birch, was to see many a happy gathering in the years to come.

It was Janet who christened it, "the house that Jack built", and as Jack had promised, we were living in it before freeze-up.

After surviving the cold winter gales, snug and cozy in our lovely new home, I one day received an official-looking document.

It was a letter from the planning commission telling me that I could build the house!

Chapter
Twenty-eight

The Indian people are a constant cause for puzzlement to their white neighbors, and those closest to them – generally ranchers – are often as puzzled by them as any city dwellers. They are looked upon with distant affection mixed, sometimes, with disdain.

There is often an impatience toward them, and this is not always justifiable, for sometimes white men do not understand their psychology or their culture. There is a reluctance on the part of the older people to have the children educated solely in the white man's ways and if the Plains Indians are often dour and don't smile easily, perhaps it's because they don't have much to smile about.

Janet and I often felt sorry for them and wished we could go beyond medicine to help them in a society that was either too patronizing, too indifferent, or even threatening.

Reserves are perhaps spacious enough, but they are not pleasure resorts. The Indian who leaves his, or her, reserve enters a strange and sometimes frightening world, almost always a degrading world. On the reserves a few of them live in reasonably modern homes, but large numbers live in shacks, often without running water or plumbing. On the other hand, at the first sign of summer they are likely to forsake their ramshackle homes and set up their tepees nearby. This may be preferable for a number of good reasons. But then, it seems that some Indians have lost their camping skills.

One Indian complained to me that during a rainstorm, water had flooded the floor of his tepee.

"Why didn't you dig a ditch all round it?" I asked, remembering my own camping days, when I had dealt with many a potential flood on the hills and moors of my native Scotland.

"I've never heard of that, boss," I was told by a poker-faced Stony. I have never been sure that I wasn't being kidded, for the sudden torrential downpours that occur in Alberta would need, not shallow ditches, but deep trenches to contain them.

A friend of mine, trusted by the Indians, was present when one of our eminent politicians was ceremonially made an honorary chief of one of the Alberta tribes. Being made a chief can be as encouraging to the natural pomposity of some people as receiving a directorship in a bank. Being made a chief is a subtly sought-after honor for some reason, much favored by politicians, and Indians, who are not at all fools, can sometimes be cajoled into conferring this distinction upon our legislators.

The great man received his Indian name, translatable into "Great White Wind". No doubt in the course of the ceremony he delivered a ringing address on the natural nobility of his impassive listeners. The rites of the ceremony completed, and the tom-toms silenced, he left without a glance at the rural slum around him.

It was after his departure that the elders, as elegant in their own way in their buckskins and feathers as any potentate of Empire (some of whom wear ostrich feathers in their own dress hats), broke into cackles of laughter. They slapped one another on the back, laughing in a most undignified and un-Indian way.

It transpired that in their Indian tongue there are nuances of meaning in the words. "Great White Wind" had a number of variables, some of them associated with the necessary intestinal functions of living. To his dying day, the Great Man never knew of the joke that had been played upon him. It was a private affair.

The Indian sense of humor, like that of the Scots, has a sly and flinty quality to it. Perhaps that is why the Scots have got on so well with the native peoples.

Janet, Catriona and I were driving through a remote area of Northern Ontario once when I realized that, with long distances between service stations, I should fill my gasoline tank as soon as possible. We came to a lonely filling station. I stopped the car beside the pump. There was no response, although the garage lights were on, so I opened the door and entered. A large man wearing overalls eventually appeared, wiping his greasy hands on a greasier cloth.

"Yeah. What d'you want?"

"I need petrol," I told him.

"Petrol?" he repeated, "petrol?"

Suddenly I realized that, without thinking, I had reverted to the almost forgotten terminology of England.

"Oh!" I said. "I'm sorry, I mean gasoline."

"Ah! gasoline," repeated the garageman. "Gasoline. Now you're talking. Where do you come from?"

"Scotland."

The man stopped, looked me up and down as if I had descended from outer space, and without a word, bellowed into the garage.

"Joe! Come out here."

Joe came out. On top of his overalls he wore a heavy lumber jacket. He was even larger than his companion.

"This guy says he's Scotch," said the first man to his friend.

"I *am* Scotch," I assured him, and then somewhat taken aback by their continued appraisal, I added, "Haven't you two guys ever seen a Scotsman before?"

"Well," said Joe, "Since you mention it, we haven't. Hell, this place is full of McNeils and MacLeods – but they're all bloody Indians. You're the first *real* Scotchman we've ever seen."

Razor Tooth was no mixture. He was a pure blood Indian. Raven-haired, with a wrinkled mahogany-complexioned face in which black eyes looked upon the world with impassive watchfulness, Razor nevertheless had a quiet, pawky sense of humor. He had fought in the Canadian Army in the First World War, and had no qualms about mixing with white men. Indeed it was rumored that old comrades kept him so well supplied with liquor that he was able to run a thriving and of course quite illegal bootlegging business on certain of the reservations in Southern Alberta. It may all have been gossip, for Razor, if a suspect, somehow eluded apprehension by the men of the Royal Canadian Mounted, one of whom, a corporal at High River, was that gem – a policeman who in the face of adversity could retain his sense of humor, as well as a sneaking affection for his adversary.

"Razor, y'old bugger," the corporal remarked banteringly one day as he came across the Indian loafing in High River's Medicine Tree Park, "why can't you find some honest work t'do."

"Why should I do that, cop'l?"

161

"Well – it would earn you some decent, honest money for a change."

"What'd I do with it, cop'l?"

"You could save it, you old sinner."

"An' then what?"

"Why! – when you're old you could sit in the sun and enjoy life."

"Boss," said Razor in that soft way the Indians talk, "Ah'm not workin' now – an' Ah'm sittin' in the sun enjoyin' myself now."

Defeated once again, the corporal retreated, leaving the philosopher to his thoughts.

It was the same philosopher who, upon reading the headlines in a daily newspaper, turned to a man in High River. "Read that," he commanded.

"What about it?" was the reply. "It just says: 'More Married Women Going Out to Work'."

"That's right," replied our philosopher. "It just proves one thing. White man finally wising up."

Twenty years later, I met Razor at the entrance to the Morley Reserve. He must have been over eighty then, old, bent, and failing, but when I asked him where he wanted to go, he replied,

"Cochrane. The hotel."

I dropped him off just outside the hotel in the center of town.

"Thanks, boss," and then, "could you lend me five dollars till next week, doc?"

I settled for one, which is what he expected, and admonished him, "Now, Razor, don't spend it all on liquor."

He stopped, looked at me and said, "Ah'll have t'spend it all on liquor. At my age what else *can* y'spend it on?"

Within a few weeks he had gone to meet a Greater Philosopher at the Great Pow-wow in the Sky, and there, I hope, he sits in the sun enjoying himself.

Chapter
Twenty-nine

We had just finished in the operating room. The last patient of the morning's "list" quietly coming out of the anesthetic was "in recovery" next door and we three doctors, still dressed in our O.R. greens, were helping ourselves to coffee in the staff room.

My friend, Dr. Andrew Little, was already at work, dictating the details of his surgical procedures. The second member of the trio was stretched out on the couch. I had "assisted" at all three cases we had done that morning – the removal of a gall bladder, a hernia repair, and some more minor procedure. It had been no strain for me. I couldn't say the same for my two colleagues. As surgeon and anesthetist they had faced their responsibilities. I had put on clamps where and when needed. I had occasionally ligatured or secured a bleeding vessel. I had attempted to anticipate the surgeon's every move and make his field of vision clearer by either holding large retractors steadily in place while he worked or by undertaking some other maneuvers. Sometimes I had succeeded in these endeavors. But I had occasionally been told to get my unmentionable hand out of the way before it was clamped to the gall bladder. Altogether it had been, for me, a pleasantly relaxed morning. I had spent it in the company of two men I liked and admired. True, it had once or twice been suggested that as a surgical assistant I possessed all the adroitness of a mentally retarded plumber's helper, but I was used to this badinage and in the best of humors with myself and my colleagues. Then someone said,

"What we need around here is another anesthetist. One day we'll get caught with nobody to give an anesthetic."

Suddenly I became aware that my friends' thoughtful gazes were directed at me.

"Don't look at me, chaps," I said. "Sure, in straightforward emergencies I've given the odd anesthetic, but that doesn't make me an anesthetist."

"How right he is," murmured Andrew, looking up from his dictating machine, "and odd couldn't be a better descriptive term. But he could be trained, you know. I really believe," he went on, "that he could be trained, although it would take untold patience on the part of his instructors."

And so, a few weeks later, I reported to the chief of anesthesiology at Calgary's Holy Cross Hospital. The medical superintendent had listened to my tale with understanding, and had put in a good word for me. Years later, as head of Family Medicine at Calgary University medical school, I would be able to recall with pride that in company with the Professor of Anesthetics, I had been instrumental, at least partly, in setting up a diploma course for young doctors going into country practice. It would take six months of their time. I knew few of them who objected to it, and many who were grateful. With their diplomas in anesthetics after six months of intensive study, these young physicians were safe anesthetists for routine procedures.

My apprenticeship now was to be a crash one, with specific and limited objectives. It was to be hoped I could be declared "safe" to give anesthetics for the kinds of operations routinely done in smaller hospitals.

Today, the specialist in anesthetics undertakes several years of intensive post-graduate training. It was not always so. In Great Britain, in my student days, anesthetists were usually known with cynical and affectionate disdain as "rag and bottle men". This soubriquet arose from the old, unsophisticated methods of rendering patients unconscious enough to be operated on. Patients lucky enough to be in the hands of an enlightened anesthetist might be given a little morphine before being wheeled into the operating room. Then, half asleep, they didn't share the experience of the less fortunate.

Many a time I have seen the latter, wide awake, terrified, brought in on hospital stretchers, surrounded by the gowned and masked figures of the operating room staff, helped to move from the trolley on to the operating table. Once there, the "rag and bottle man" appeared at the head of the operating table, placed an anesthetic mask over the patient's face, and began to pour the anesthetic – ether or chloroform – drop by drop from a piece of gauze inserted in the stopper of the bottle. Inevitably, despite reassurances, urgings, and sometimes swearing, patients struggled and fought, desperately trying to tear the mask away, pleading for "just another breath of air" until finally the struggles grew weaker and the anesthetic prevailed. It was a primitive way of doing things.

Today, "anesthetics" is almost a science – almost, but not quite, for like everything else in medicine and surgery, the human factor remains. The anesthetist must still deal with people, whose personalities, fears, idiosyncracies and physical characteristics make them all uniquely dissimilar.

While surgeons belong to one of the "glamor classes" of my profession, facing decisions that often they alone can make, the anesthetists must also show dexterity, skill and an ability to think and act, sometimes very quickly indeed. Gone are the days when the surgeons stood by, impatiently waiting for the struggles of the patient to cease so that they might operate. Today, anesthetists sit beside their patients surrounded by a battery of sophisticated equipment and they will tell the surgeon when he may arrange his sterile drapes and make that first incision. Only when the anesthetist "gives the nod" will the surgeon proceed. Indeed, in some cases the anesthetist may (if there is any doubt of the patient's ability to withstand the operation) advise against surgery altogether, and it would be a foolhardy surgeon who refused to listen.

The anesthetists' task is to see their patients through their operation: to assess their psychological and physical health beforehand, to "put them to sleep", to take care of them during surgery and to be responsible for them for usually 24 hours post-operatively. It is an immense, and sometimes a hair-raising responsibility.

Specialist anesthetists have at their fingertips a variety of techniques, a long "in depth" training in the normal and abnormal aspects of respiratory and cardiac action, and they will be able to anesthetize patients during prolonged and complicated operations.

My objectives, as I began my crash course, were much more simple. Wisely, I was instructed in a few techniques and methods of anesthesia. I was urged to master them, and acquire a sound knowledge of the drugs to be used. My instructors patiently stood over me as I worked. In the beginning I was allowed to control already anesthetized patients during their operation. From this humble start I was eventually promoted and allowed to anesthetize patients, again under supervision. So I progressed, passing from supervised supervision of an unconscious patient, to induction, intubation and solo care. Then one morning, my tutor said casually,

"Go ahead. If you need me I'll be in the doctors' room" (an annex of the operating room). I had arrived.

More supervision followed, more tuition, but one day I was told I was "safe" to give anesthetics for most of the operations we might undertake.

In carrying out his examination of the patient prior to surgery, the anesthetist must inquire into any history of illness that might be relevant or allergies that might affect the anesthesia. Then, the night before surgery, a mild tranquilizer ensures a sound sleep, and an hour or so prior to the operation, a smaller dose of a tranquilizer is given so that the patient arrives in the operating room – it is hoped – blissfully unaware or uncaring – of the impending procedure. Medicine and surgery being inexact sciences, this ideal is not always achieved.

Once in the operating room with the intravenous "drip" in place in the patient's arm, the anesthetist makes a final check of his apparatus. Is the oxygen flowing freely and on demand? Are all equipment valves functioning smoothly? Is "the drip" flowing freely into the selected vein? Is the patient "in good shape"? Specifically, have all his or her false teeth been removed? Are there any impediments to a safe airway? Is the patient correctly and safely positioned on the operating table?

These, and other details attended to, the anesthetist puts the patient to sleep. A hypnotic sedative drug is slowly inserted into the plastic tubing of the intravenous drip and the already dreamy patient is asked to count to ten. With skill, and a little bit of luck, that number is never reached. Quiet, regular breathing indicates success. The patient has lost consciousness. Quickly the hypnotic is followed by the injection of a second drug that renders the respiratory muscles of the throat flaccid and a tube is passed down into the breathing canal. This procedure, known as intubation, must quickly be accomplished and the intubating tube immediately connected to the apparatus conveying the correct quantities of anesthetic and oxygen. For the duration of the operation it will be the anesthetist's duty to superintend the patient's breathing and whole physical well-being. The breathing might be normal or assisted; if the latter, the anesthetist gently propels the correct mixture of oxygen and anesthetic into the patient's lungs at regular intervals. The anesthetist must also watch for any alteration in the heart, respiratory rate or blood pressure and be prepared to take appropriate action where necessary. Above all, it would be a foolhardy anesthetist who did not look regularly at the color of the patient's blood as the surgeon operates, for bright red blood means a good oxygen supply to heart and brain, and dark red, the reverse and danger.

The operation completed, it remains the duty of the anesthetist to supervise the patient's safe recovery in the immediate post-operative period.

I gave anesthetics for years. I loved the challenge, became competent, was accepted by my colleagues, warily perhaps at first, but increasingly as time went by. With care, and as always with a little bit of luck, my anesthetics went well, and a great day arrived when, after a difficult operation, a visiting specialist said I had given "an elegant anesthetic". What praise from the gods!

Nowhere is the power of positive suggestion more useful than in the field of anesthesia. Many people are deadly afraid of being put to sleep, despite today's statistics which show anesthetics capably given to be, in the great majority of cases, safe procedures. Nevertheless, that fear of the unknown remains. The rapport established between anesthetist and patient – usually strangers to one another – is very important indeed. That preliminary interview and assessment can work wonders for the patient's mental well-being.

I had made it my custom, whenever possible, to drop in on patients the night before surgery. A short chat always seemed to be welcomed. However, I often used a variant of hypnotic technique, teaching patients to relax and showing them how easy it can be to "drift into sleep" just with the aid of suggestion. My little visits helped to relax tense people, and in the morning I would often find my patient responding to a quite small dose of intravenous pentothal, the hypnotic drug we used to induce sleep; and that was a benefit in itself.

So when I was asked to give Mrs. McVey, a stranger to me, the anesthetic for her gall bladder surgery, I appeared the evening before, examined her and sat by her bedside for my usual introductory chat. We got on well together and in the course of our conversation she told me how her husband and she ran a herd of Black Angus cattle. Now I had learned a bit about cattle over the years, but I was no expert. Herefords, with their brown and white markings, were everywhere and easy to spot, but Galloways and Angus, both Scottish breeds, were black and I was never quite sure which was which. But Mrs. McVey was sure and she waxed enthusiastic over the virtues of her Angus herd.

Came the morning and I appeared, as usual, that ten or fifteen minutes before the surgeons, to check my patient, my equipment, and to have my patient fast asleep and ready for the operation. But not this morning. Mrs. McVey was wide awake. There could be any number of reasons for this, apprehension being one of them, for some drugs which normally sedate can sometimes stimulate quite unexpectedly and it seemed to me that Mrs. McVey was very wide awake indeed.

In my best bedside manner I soothed her. Around me all was bustle. The lights of the operating room emphasized the whiteness of the wall tiles against the dark green of our sterile drapes. Bowls were being placed in readiness for the operation. Instruments were being checked. Surgical swabs were being counted and counted again. The nurses were bustling about the operating room making sure that all was ready.

Mrs. McVey's anxiety was as obvious to them as it was to me and so I decided to reassure my charge by introducing her to "the girls". They, knowing my little ways, responded. Each nurse found time to stop for that second or two and bid our patient a cheery "good morning", thus implying that this was just another routine morning and that our patient simply had nothing to worry about.

I set up my drip, found a good vein in her forearm, inserted the needle, saw that the intravenous fluid was dripping freely, then inserted into the plastic tubing the syringe containing the pentothal. The time had come to initiate the anesthetic. As the pentothal slowly entered the blood stream, my patient would go quietly to sleep.

That is the theory. Usually it works. But Mrs. McVey was showing no inclination to cooperate. She was watching my every move. Chattering reassuringly to her, I began,

"Now Mrs. McVey, just count from one to ten, slowly."

Confident that my patient would never get to double digits, I quietly injected the pentothal.

"Eleven – twelve," she intoned, those Scottish eyes of hers intently fixed on that needle.

"Just keep going, m'dear," I said, perhaps a little testily by now. I didn't like to use one drop more of any drug than I needed to.

That concentrated stare remained undimmed.

Distract her attention, I thought. Talk about her consuming interest. She raises cattle, one breed superb, the other just all right. And then suddenly I thought, but which lot was hers? Black Galloway or Black Angus? Angus, or was it Galloway? For the life of me I couldn't remember.

Distract her attention. That's the very thing.

"Ladies," I said to my preoccupied colleagues, "have you ever seen Mrs. McVey's cattle? She's got the most splendid herd of Galloways you've every seen."

Suddenly, her head was raised from the pillow.

"Galloways?" she declared in her wrath. "Galloways? We keep Black Angus, I'll have you know. It's a poor kind of a Scotsman – it's a poor kind of a Scotsman," she repeated, "that can't tell the difference between Galloway and Angus cattle."

Then immediately – and thank goodness, forgetfully, she went to sleep.

Chapter
Thirty

Monica was our secretary. She liked working with people more than with test tubes and was a discreet employee with that sixth sense that anticipates trouble, even in a telephone conversation.

"It's Mr. and Mrs. Jamieson to see you," she said. "They're your last patients for the day, and," she added, "they look upset, so you might want to spend a bit of time with them. In fact, I let a few people come before them so you could do that if you wanted to."

Looking up from my notes, I nodded, perhaps a little questioningly, in answer to her statement. The Jamiesons were ushered in, and sat side by side on the settee beside my desk.

I liked them. Bill Jamieson was a clean-cut, intelligent man in his late thirties, the kind of fellow who looked you straight in the eye when he spoke. He was a carpenter and seldom out of work, for employers were only too happy to have such a capable workman. Joan Jamieson was a few years younger than her husband, and in a quiet, self-effacing way, she was a pretty woman. Like a lot of those "prairie women" there was an elegance, a quality about her, a kind of quiet dignity. Their three children, the youngest a toddler, completed the family, and a warm, united one it was.

Monica had been right in her assessment. Anxiety showed in the tight lines around Jamieson's mouth, and his eyes met mine unsmilingly as my glance passed from one to the other. I wasted no time on pleasantries.

"Tell me. What's worrying you two?"

Bill glanced sideways at his wife, half nodding his head in her direction.

"It's Joan, doctor. She should speak to you about a problem she has. I hope you don't mind my coming in with her, but I'm as worried as she is."

"She's your wife, Bill. Sharing problems is the name of the game if you care – or can talk to one another. So tell me . . ."

"I've got a lump in my breast." Joan Jamieson's apprehension

170

was obvious. "It's probably me just fussing – but would you look at it?" She was struggling to remain composed and I looked at her encouragingly.

"No woman should ever need to say she's fussing about any lump in her breast. When did you first notice it? A month ago? – a week ago – how long? Approximately will do."

"It's a month or two. Maybe more. I tried to ignore it at first. It didn't seem to be anything, but I know it's got bigger."

There was no point in beating about the bush. While she undressed in the examining room next door, I spoke to her husband.

"Any lump in a breast should be analyzed. Many are simple cysts, but that's not the point. A diagnosis must be established scientifically. Now I'll give you a preliminary opinion, and sometimes that can be pretty exact – but I think she's probably going to be seen by a specialist, and soon, too. A proper diagnosis is vital!" I emphasized the point as I made for the examining room.

I had developed that conviction as a result of hard experience. Some years before I'd been visited by another lady. She had just come to the area and only wanted to introduce herself to me, she said, in case she needed to call on me at some future date. She, too, had a lump in her breast, but she told me, smiling brightly, there was simply no need to examine it that day. She had seen a specialist in Eastern Canada only a month before, and he had assured her that the lump was a simple one.

What had he done in the way of examination, I wanted to know? Had he X-rayed her, withdrawn any fluid for examination?

"Oh," said my new patient, "he examined it carefully and said it was just a simple cyst. He didn't need to do any X-rays or take it out, or anything like that. He said there wasn't any need for me to worry."

I wasn't impressed by the specialist's opinion but I checked his qualifications. They were real enough. Three months later when she came back for a "check-up", I examined that hard, malignant mass with horror. The tragedy that ensued might have been avoided had the specialist done adequate tests in the first place – and had I insisted on doing a repeat examination when she came to my office on that introductory visit, as was my moral duty.

I was going to make no such error in my examination of Mrs. Jamieson.

The answer was only too easy. The lump, though small, was hard, craggy and adherent to the overlying skin. The nipple was being pulled slightly to one side. A third year medical student would have understood the ominous significance of those signs.

Joan Jamieson's eyes were searching my face.

"It's cancer, isn't it, doctor? I can see it in your eyes."

"It could be," I began cautiously, waiting for the tears I knew would come. "It could be. So we're going to get it removed and analyzed. That's the only way to be sure. Meantime, I'm going to let Dr. Janet have a look."

I knew what that lady's opinion would be, but while she talked to Mrs. Jamieson, I explained matters to her husband.

Joan Jamieson was seen within days by an excellent surgeon who quickly had her admitted to the Calgary General. There, the growth's malignancy was confirmed, and a radical removal of the breast performed. At the conclusion of the operation the surgeon phoned my office.

"It's cancer, of course. Unfortunately it's a malignant type and there's been invasion of the axillary glands. I'm sorry to have to say it, but the outlook is anything but good."

Advances in chemotherapy and radiology have made the post-operative care of many kinds of cancer a much more optimistic affair than it was twenty years ago, but I had no cause for optimism in Joan Jamieson's case. Even at operation, the surgeon knew the cancer had spread.

Our duty was to give moral support through what is a harrowing time for women, when they not only face a bleak future, but often feel that the femininity that attracted their husbands to them has been destroyed. There can be a feeling of physical rejection, of great mental hurt.

We sent Joan Jamieson to the Calgary Cancer Clinic where, even in the 1950s, the most up-to-date treatment was provided free to cancer sufferers by an enlightened government. Their report, supported by the findings of the surgeon's biopsy, confirmed our worst fears. The cancer had spread and, but for a miracle, was beyond control.

Mrs. Jamieson's condition gradually deteriorated, almost imperceptibly at first, but more rapidly as the months went by. It was perhaps a year after the operation that Bill Jamieson, his quiet desperation only too obvious, told us that he wanted to transfer his wife to a clinic in the United States. He laid his stetson on the desk top as he spoke.

"We know you're doing all you can, doc, but *I* have to do something. She's just fading away before my eyes. I can't stand to see her like this. Surely, there's somewhere else, some specialist somewhere . . .?"

How often every doctor hears desperate parents, husbands or wives utter those words!

Grimly I shook my head.

"No, Bill. She's seen excellent people. Alberta spares no expense in treating such cases. But I know how you feel, and if you want to go to the States to get an opinion, that's fine. Some of the greatest clinics in the world are there. We've sent quite a few people to the Mayo Clinic. I'll be happy to phone them. Their fees are always reasonable too, and you'd come away knowing you've seen some of the best people anywhere in North America. I'll arrange it all."

Life can be a very cruel business. Who could have blamed Bill Jamieson for wanting to take his wife to some famous, far-distant hospital? All the same, I was not prepared for what was to follow.

He reached into the pocket of his blue jeans, produced a brochure, and laid it on the desk before me.

"That's where I want to take her. They're working miracles with cancer cases there – even the hopeless ones. Just read it, doc. I only wish I'd heard of this outfit before."

If there was a trace of hurt or remonstrance in his voice or the look he gave me, I hardly noticed it as I studied the folder. The glossy prints showed green lawns and attractive haciendas silhouetted against the blue skies and warm desert sun of the Southern United States. The clinic's specialist in charge stood by a hospital bed set on the lawn. A pretty nurse stood beside him. From the bed a delicate-looking, yet appealingly beautiful invalid smiled gratefully at the white-coated physician in charge. He was a man apparently somewhere in his sixties. Beaming

173

benevolently on the world through his gold-rimmed spectacles, here was the very picture of a kindly, yet authoritarian healer.

And that, according to the expensively-produced brochure, was exactly what he was. In cases that had defied the most brilliant of medical minds, he had succeeded.

Urging Jamieson not to make any hasty moves, I promised to make inquiries. I telephoned the registrar of the College of Physicians and Surgeons. This official controls the right and wrong doings of his colleagues in practice, and he might, I thought, know of this particular clinic. He did!

The clinic was registered with no health authority that existed. Complaints had already been made against it, particularly with regard to its extortionate charges. And "the specialist" was not a member of any known medical or any other professional register. Despite his distinguished appearance, his exotic surroundings, and his self-styled titles, he was a quack!

I told Jamieson the results of my inquiries. I urged him to go to some University clinic and offered to expedite such an appointment. I sensed his growing antagonism. His whole attitude suggested I had not helped before. How could I help now?

He took his wife to the clinic described in the brochure, despite my warnings, and in the end I realized the futility of trying to stop him. Anyone might have done the same under the circumstances. But I offered to write to "the specialist". My letter, written as if to a colleague, contained all the details of the treatment prescribed and given by the Calgary Cancer Clinic, as well as a summary of the surgeon's sinister findings. I spent a good deal of time in composing that letter. It was a masterpiece of diplomacy, I thought.

"Mr. Jamieson," I ended, "is a working man of limited means. In the circumstances, I would appeal to you, once you have assessed my patient's condition, to return her immediately to the care of the Alberta Government's cancer clinic."

I didn't see him for some months after that. I did hear a few reports. Joan Jamieson had been admitted to the clinic as an emergency case on her arrival. As the weeks passed, I was told, she was showing signs of steady improvement. The success of the new treatment was indeed miraculous.

When I met Jamieson one day in the street, his greeting was coldly courteous.

Yes, indeed, his wife was steadily improving. No, she was still losing weight, but that was due to the improper treatment she had received at the hands of myself and the provincial cancer clinic. Weight loss was to be expected, was temporary, and rapid improvement was expected shortly.

Had the "specialist" read my letter, I wanted to know. Yes he had and was very angry about it, for if Mrs. Jamieson had been sent to him at the very outset, she'd be better off now. As it was, only prolonged care in the other clinic would put right the harm that had been done. Coldly, Jamieson nodded to me and walked away.

Several months elapsed and I heard that Mrs. Jamieson had come home. She was being treated "long distance" from the clinic. The "specialist", still confident of her eventual recovery, was sending her regular supplies of special pills. The trouble was that they were unobtainable in Canada. They were specially made in Bulgaria or India. They were also extremely expensive, a hundred or two dollars for a few weeks' supply. But they were, wrote the "specialist", Joan Jamieson's one hope of survival.

It couldn't go on, of course. A few weeks before her death I was told that their home had been sold to pay the clinic's expenses. But not a word of complaint came from Bill Jamieson. He had spent his all for the woman he loved.

I met him some time afterwards. His once handsome face was lined and gaunt. Bitterly, he walked past me without speaking.

A month or two later, the clinic hit the headlines. It had been closed by order of the United States Government.

But the story had not quite ended. The "specialist" simply moved out of the United States to a sunnier climate. His clinic was soon in business again, under another name. No doubt the "specialist" charged a little more for the extra sunshine, and the inconvenience to which he had been subjected.

Chapter
Thirty-one

I had been practising in Okotoks for over ten years. I had delivered Johnny Blakenay in my first year there and had dealt with his childhood diseases. Now he was returning my glances impassively. I kept looking at him as I listened to his mother's reasons for keeping her offspring from school that morning and bringing him to see me instead.

Johnny hadn't been feeling well since the previous evening. He wouldn't eat, which was unusual for him, and he had stomach ache and diarrhea. It wasn't a very alarming story. Mrs. Blakenay was a cheerful, sensitive woman in her thirties, and if she was worried about Johnny, the chances were that she had reason to be, so, when her catalogue of his symptoms was completed, I turned to him.

"That's about it, Johnny, eh? Nothing else?"

Johnny was ten, a smaller replica of his father, a stocky, polite but laconic farmer, and already he was showing signs of developing the same skills as his dad, as well. Although he was smaller than the rest of his classmates, Johnny excelled in sports, just as his father had.

I had watched him play in the Okotoks Pee-Wee hockey team against other small boys. The ice rinks are institutions in many prairie towns. Huge barn-like structures, often unheated, the ice formed by water poured onto the floor and allowed to freeze for the duration of the winter, the rinks are often one of the focal points of community life during the cold months. Crowds of spectators gather for the various games. Partisanship is usually good-natured, with much clanging of cow bells and vociferous advice to the players and, of course, the referees. Muffled to the eyebrows in warm clothing of variegated colors, it may be "30 below" outside, but the hockey crowds keep themselves and the atmosphere in the rink warm, often in more ways than one.

The principal team locally, the Okotoks Oilers, competed for the championship of the "Big Six" League, but the country teams were not ignored. Neither were the small boys, and it was at a Pee-Wee game that I had first noticed Master Blakenay.

Johnny was different. When a goal was scored by himself or by one of his side he didn't join in the customary mild hysteria of hugging, helmet clapping and bottom patting indulged in by Canada's famous teams. He would quietly skate backwards, away from his exuberant team-mates and take his place for the impending face-off, dourly ready for the next business on hand. Johnny was already very much his own man.

And now he sat in my office, watching me just as I was watching him.

"That's about it, then, Johnny?" I repeated. "Have you thrown up?"

"Nope."

"How d'you feel?"

"Not good."

You couldn't have said it was a flowing conversation and so I decided to send him into the examination room, told him to strip off, and lie on the examination couch.

I began by just looking at his breathing and his abdomen. Nothing there – just a serious-faced small boy watching me. Then I palpated his abdomen using little pressure at first, then pressing deeper from one quadrant of the abdomen to another and from left to right. I watched his face as I examined him and it seemed to me that he grimaced just a little as I pressed on his abdomen on the right side.

"Where does it hurt, Johnny, when I press in?"

"Everywhere."

"Does it hurt a lot?"

"Nope."

I repeated my examination; again that tightening of the facial muscles, and again that denial of pain. In my judgment, young Blakenay was something of a stoic. It was a weakness to admit to pain and he wasn't going to do it. That is all very well, but stoicism isn't a very good diagnostic aid.

Despite his attack of diarrhea I suspected an underlying acute appendicitis. Appendicitis can occasionally be accompanied or obscured by diarrhea, and it's all too easy to make a mistake. I had made that mistake once. More by good luck than any skill

177

on my part, catastrophe had been averted and I had no intention of repeating my error, which has been made by many a better man than me.

My memories took me back to my days as a medical student. I was twenty-two years old at the time, and a final year student in the wards of Sir Archibald Young, Regius professor of surgery at Glasgow. It was there that I first saw how difficult it can be to diagnose this still dangerous condition.

Sir Archibald (or "Archie" as he was clandestinely called by the student body) must have been the last professor at Glasgow University Medical School to wear a frock coat. He was a small, quiet man, slim, elderly, grey-haired, but his usually serious face could be transformed by his smile. His morning rounds of the wards were great occasions, as, accompanied by the ward sister, he made his way from bed to bed followed by his retinue of assistant professors, occasional distinguished visitors, lecturers, nurses and medical students, the latter standing on tiptoe at the periphery of the crowd, straining their ears lest they miss what the great man might say.

He had the reputation of being a demanding chief and a strict disciplinarian. Only a fool would apply for a position in his wards, I was told by several of my cronies. However, I speedily discovered not only that Sir Archibald had a quiet, pawky sense of humor, but that he was always interested in the young and their opinions. When he considered it necessary he also had a courteous disregard for the rigid protocols of professional ethics and manners that sometimes bedeviled our profession. And that disregard taught me a lesson I never forgot.

One night when I was the student on duty, a Dr. Sutherland phoned from the poverty-stricken Gorbals area of Glasgow. He wanted to send in a child he suspected of having an acutely inflamed appendix. He had, he said, spoken to Sir Archibald about the case.

A bed was found, the child admitted and examined immediately by the surgical specialist on duty. His examination was meticulous and as I stood beside him he delineated the various diagnostic possibilities. He eventually said with great finality,

"This is a case of simple gastroenteritis," prescribed a fluid diet with bed rest overnight and left me to compile the case notes.

An hour had elapsed when, busy at my tasks, I saw the charge nurse hurriedly rise to her feet as Professor Young entered, his tailcoat flapping rhythmically as he strolled up the ward, his hands clasped together behind him underneath the flaps of his old-fashioned coat.

He walked toward me and remarked,

"You've had a case sent in by Dr. Sutherland?"

"Yes sir," I replied. "It's been seen by Dr. So-and-So," naming one of Sir Archie's subordinates. "It's a case of simple enteritis."

"Sutherland's an old colleague of mine," said the chief, "and very experienced. If Sutherland suspects an appendicitis, he's likely to be right. I think I'll have a look for myself."

"But, sir," I hastened to say, "the patient's already been seen by Dr. So-and-So, and he says it's a simple diarrhea!"

I stood in much greater awe of that particular surgeon than I did of the chief himself and I think the latter knew that, for he turned to me. There was an amused twinkle in his eyes.

"Is that so?" he asked. "But you'll have no objection, Gibson, if I look at the child?"

"Oh no, sir!" I hastily assured him.

"And you'll accompany me?"

"Oh yes, sir."

"That is most obliging of you, my boy," replied the Regius professor without the hint of a smile on his face.

So I led Sir Archie up that long many-bedded ward to see the newcomer. Silently he examined the child.

"I'm going to do a rectal examination," he announced as he sent me off for a surgical glove and some lubricant cream. "A rectal examination can be the acid test in diagnosing appendicitis," he emphasized. "And it should never be omitted."

Gently he inserted his gloved finger into the child's anus. If his examining finger could reach the area of an inflamed appendix, its pressure on the pelvic floor might produce pain.

"Nothing," he said finally, as the child experienced no discomfort. But still he was not satisfied. He leaned over the child's face and sniffed his breath. He turned to me.

"Come here, boy," he commanded.

He gently propelled my face close to the little fellow's mouth. "Smell his breath," he said.

I sniffed. Sir Archie's hand drew me gently upright.

"What did that smell remind you of?"

"I don't know, sir."

"Smell it again, then," and down went my head again, my shoulder still in Sir Archie's grasp.

"I don't know, sir," I admitted as he drew me upright.

"It is the smell of rotten apples," said Sir Archie. "Isn't it?"

"Yes, sir."

"Smell it again," commanded my interrogator relentlessly. "Breathe out – and smell again." And down went my head once more.

"Never forget that smell, my boy," said Professor Young, "for it is the smell of a gangrenous appendix. I shall operate immediately."

Watched by an intensely interested group of students (for I had quickly told some of my colleagues of the difference of opinion between the two specialists), the professor removed an appendix that was grey with gangrene.

Many a competent surgeon has "missed" an appendix. In the old days before the antibiotics this meant, at best, weeks of illness and a long recuperation. Often patients died. Dealing with an acute appendix can still be a difficult problem. It can be an easy or a difficult diagnosis to make, just as the operation can be easy or very difficult. In the old days the decision largely rested on the doctor's skill as a clinical diagnostician, on his "feel", experience, clinical instinct. Today there are many clinical tests that help the physician to make an early and accurate diagnosis, but with the appendix, the old adage, "if in doubt, take it out," should always be at the back of the doctor's mind.

But many years later in Okotoks, Johnny Blakenay, even with all those tests to help in making a decision, was still a puzzle. I admitted him to hospital for observation. His blood count remained normal and if my suspicions were correct his white cell count should have been raised. So should his pulse rate and temperature. Stolidly he told me he had no pain when I did a rectal examination. There was just that slight tenderness on his abdomen when I pushed. Even his diarrhea had settled down.

I called one of my colleagues into consultation. He agreed with my decision. "Masterly inactivity" was called for. Johnny should stay in hospital, have the tests repeated and be allowed only limited fluids by mouth.

Still vaguely uneasy about him, I went to the hospital late in the evening. Johnny was as uncomplaining as ever, but this time I decided upon action.

I phoned my colleague of the morning. He was out of town for the evening. I phoned Dr. Andrew Little, at Nanton, a town thirty miles or so south of Okotoks. Would he come up, I asked. I wanted to remove a child's appendix. It was an unwritten rule that while a consultation was a matter for discussion, a decision to operate was final, and shortly my friend appeared in the doctors' room at the hospital. Dr. Little is a widely respected surgeon and while, over the years, I had mastered a variety of emergency procedures, I always had greater peace of mind when he was in the operating room with me.

He made no demur about my decision to remove young Blakenay's appendix and speedily we began the operation, making the incision just above the usual site of the caecum, the small sac of bowel from which the appendix is suspended. Gently we picked up the peritoneum (the inner membrane that lines the abdomen), and opened into the abdominal cavity.

But the caecum was not in its usual place. It lay high in the abdomen, which perhaps explained why our patient experienced no pain on rectal examination. I had thought that Johnny's ingrained stoicism had been responsible for his refusal to admit to pain. Perhaps I was misled by my own assessment of that little character's toughness. No doubt stoicism had played its part but when he said he felt no pain over the appendix area, he was right. The appendix wasn't *in* the appendix area. It was tucked away elsewhere – and that sometimes happens, just to add to all the other difficulties associated with what is too often dismissed as a straightforward complaint.

When the caecum was exposed with the appendix lying behind it, the appendix was inflamed, and its tip showed the ominous grey of early gangrene. It was removed with the utmost care and Johnny Blakenay was safely taken to the post-operative care ward.

"Interesting case," said Andrew afterwards. "Nothing to go on really. No vomiting. Temperature and pulse hardly above normal. Not what you'd expect, considering what we found. Most unusual! Tell me – what made you decide to go in?"

"Well," I replied cautiously. "There was that right-sided tenderness all right and my instinct told me something was amiss, but the deciding factor was his breath – it smelled of rotten apples."

Chapter
Thirty-two

I liked the look of Peter Drasny when he introduced himself. He was a splendid specimen of humanity, nearly six feet tall, broad-shouldered, built like an athlete, a man somewhere in his mid-twenties. He gave an impression of quiet self-confidence as he spoke, his dark, lively eyes were watchful and yet he smiled easily, too. There was a warmth about him, and with his dark hair and sunburned complexion he was a handsome, attractive lad. When he spoke, he spoke well, using excellent English. I thought he might be a university student on vacation.

The preliminaries of introduction over, he sat down and I began.

"And now, Mr. Drasny, what can I do for you?"

"Just call me Peter, doctor. Everybody does that, and I feel happier with it that way."

"All right, Peter. That's fine with me."

"Do you remember John Driscoll?" he asked. "He's a patient of yours."

"Very well! How is he? I haven't seen John in months."

"He's been away for months. Up north, where I work. That's

where I met him. He thinks well of you. I'm staying in Calgary for two weeks," said my new patient, "and I decided to come and see you myself. You don't mind, I hope?"

"I'm delighted," I laughingly replied. "There's no better recommendation than one from a satisfied patient, you know. But tell me," I went on, "you weren't born in Canada, were you? There's just the trace of a European accent there, and I can't place it."

"I was born in Hungary," said Peter. "We left after the war when I was a little boy. My father had disappeared – taken away by the Russians, and my mother made up her mind that things would be different for me. She walked for days with me to get to the border. I remember it a bit. She carried me a lot of the way. I was often cold and hungry, and I guess so was she. I remember I cried a lot but she never complained. We hid sometimes during the day when we got near the border. She was afraid of the police, of the Russians. But we made it. We came to Canada fifteen years ago."

"And you like it?"

"Yes," he smiled quietly. "I owe a great deal to Canada. I'm making good money. I'm able to give my mother the kind of house she deserves. You see, I owe everything to my mother. I owe the freedom I have here to her. I owe my whole future to her."

He wasn't smiling anymore and I could understand the depth of emotion he felt.

"I understand, Peter, in a way, but only people who have gone through that kind of experience can really understand. But tell me, what makes you want to see a doctor?"

"You're not going to tell me I'm neurotic, I hope?"

"No, I doubt that, Peter. Telling someone they're neurotic is a diagnosis of last resort. And furthermore, there are precious few of us who haven't been neurotic about something or other at some time in our lives. So go ahead and tell me why you want to see me."

"I'm constantly tired. That's about it."

"Is this tiredness new?"

"Quite new. I've felt tired, weak for no reason I can think of, for about six months."

183

"Have you seen a doctor?"

"I've seen two. One up north in the Yukon and one in the city."

"And?"

"I trusted the doctor up north. He took a lot of time to examine me. He did a lot of tests. He X-rayed my chest. And he talked to me. He was very honest and told me he just didn't know what I had. I appreciated that. But I had to move away. I work very hard, and I had to move with my equipment, so I lost Dr. Salter."

"What do you do for a living?"

"I'm an independent contractor." He said it with quiet pride, and went on, "I started as a laborer, then I learned how to handle bulldozers and caterpillars. Now I own my own machine."

I looked at him with growing respect.

"Peter – I thought you might be a student on holiday. Do you read a lot?" I asked curiously, having listened to his precise English.

"Yes, I do. Conrad especially, but I like Conan Doyle too. You see, I intend to educate myself."

"Good for you, Peter. Go on. Tell me what happened when you moved."

"Nothing much. I just kept feeling very weak."

"How hard do you work?"

"Very hard – from morning till night most days."

"Perhaps you're working too hard!"

"No harder than last year or the year before – and I love the work."

"When did you see the second doctor, and what did he say?"

"Two weeks ago. He examined me," said Peter, "but not like Dr. Salter. He said he couldn't find anything wrong with me and that's when he told me I was neurotic. I'm not neurotic," he said quietly.

"And I don't think you are either," I replied, "so let's have you stripped and we'll begin this examination."

Like Dr. Salter, I could find nothing wrong. Peter Drasny had the physique of an athlete. His heart sounds and blood pressure were normal. There was no sugar in his urine that would have clinched a diagnosis of diabetes, a common cause of tiredness.

184

I have never forgotten the medical quip that "common things are commonest", and that day I did my best to eliminate all the ordinary ailments that might have made him tired. A preliminary examination of the central nervous system showed no abnormality. He was not anemic, his tonsils were not diseased, he had no chronic disorder that I could diagnose, and in the end I told him I could find nothing wrong."

"Neurotic after all?" asked Peter.

"No. I want to send you to a specialist friend of mine," I replied. "When do you have to go back up north?"

"I have two weeks' holiday. I'm staying with my mother in Calgary."

"Well," I said, smiling, "see a bit of life while you are there. D'you have a girl friend?"

"No one serious," replied Peter. "I'll marry when I meet the right one – and when I've paid off my mother's home – when I've bettered myself."

"Good for you, Peter. Give me a call tomorrow. I'll have things arranged for you."

I had him admitted to hospital for observation. The specialist's examination was as unrewarding as my own, but he, too, was suspicious and arranged to review Peter in a few months' time. When he did, there was no doubt as to the diagnosis. Peter Drasny had a rare, wasting disease of the central nervous system. It was a heartbreaking diagnosis to make, but the diagnosis was beyond doubt. Peter Drasny, unless there was a miracle, had only a few years to live. There was no known treatment for his complaint, no hope or comfort that could be offered.

He came to see me again. He looked the same handsome, stalwart young man that I had met a few months before, but he told me his weakness was at times profound. He was still able to work.

"Tell me," he said, "and tell me truthfully. How long have I got to go?"

"Three – four years, Peter."

"Can I make a deal with you, doctor? You know how I'm paying off my mother's home? I'm going back to work. I'm going to keep on working for as long as I'm able to. I'm to see the specialist in six months. He can't help me, but I'll go anyway.

185

When I can no longer work, can I come back to you? Could you put me in hospital and take care of me till it's all over?"

"Yes, Peter."

I had nothing to say, no comfort to offer him, though I said that miracles sometimes happened and he mustn't give up hope.

"Miracles, doctor?" He shook his head, slowly and deliberately. "There are no miracles. I'll come to you when I'm ready."

Two years passed. I had almost forgotten Peter Drasny, when one day my secretary came into my office. It was late in the afternoon, and I was alone. The girl's eyes were brimming with tears.

"It's Mr. Drasny. He can hardly stand. He says I've to tell you he's ready to go to hospital."

Quickly I made for the waiting room where Peter Drasny half sat, half lay in a chair. I wouldn't have known this haggard man.

"I worked till a week ago," he whispered, "and then I knew I could go on no longer. I've sold my machine. I've settled my affairs. You made me a promise, remember?"

I took him to the hospital. He asked for nothing except that his mother should be allowed to visit him as she wished.

His mother was a simple peasant woman. She could barely speak English. With that worn, grief-stricken face, etched in lines of work and pain emphasized by the babushka she wore, she seemed to typify all the suffering of Europe.

She would sit silently by her son, hour after hour, or wait in the corridor outside while the nurses worked with him, and there she stopped me one day.

"Get priest," she said, clutching at my sleeve. "He not want priest. Make him get priest or he go to purgatory forever." She wept silently.

"Mrs. Drasny, I'll talk to Peter."

When his mother was out of hearing, I broached the subject with him.

"Peter. Your mother desperately wants you to be seen by a priest."

"No priest, doctor. I have no time for the Church. She wants me to have the last rites of the Church. She's a devout Catholic. I'll have no priest giving me the last rites."

"Peter. It would please her. She's frantic about it."

His voice had dwindled to a whisper, but his "no" was vehement and I didn't speak to him about it again, though his mother pleaded with me to fetch a priest. She was living in her own hell, and would do so for the rest of her life unless something could be done for her, and so I went to see a priest for whom I had great respect.

Father Liever was an elderly man, close to retirement and, so some of his parishioners said, a conservative churchman, unbending and severe. I had never found him to be that and, as I expected, he listened sympathetically to my story.

"It's not Peter I'm concerned about, Father. It's his mother. She's suffering the tortures of the damned now."

"What do you suggest I do, doctor?"

"Peter is dying. He's hardly known me for two days. I know he's rejected your Church, but if you could come and maybe talk to his mother, it would help her."

"When do you want me to come?"

"Perhaps tomorrow."

That next day Peter Drasny's life began to ebb away. It was night when I went to fetch Father Liever. I apologized for the lateness of the hour, but my friend brushed my apologies aside. He carried an attaché case, and when he emerged from the doctors' room and accompanied me along the dimly lit corridor, he was dressed in the regalia of his Order. There was a kind of joy in that poor woman's face when she saw him.

While I waited some distance off, they talked and then the priest came toward me.

"I'd like to go into his room for a moment," he said. Seeing my sharp look he said gently, "I won't do or say anything you or your patient could disapprove of."

Quietly he followed me into the room. Peter, comatose, was facing away from him. The priest bowed his head, prayed voicelessly, then signified that we should leave.

Mrs. Drasny knelt and thanked my companion. For the first time in weeks I saw a kind of serenity in her features. As I drove the priest to his rectory, I voiced my thoughts.

"I hope I didn't involve you in something that might trouble you, Father."

"And why should it trouble me?" he asked. "I have not betrayed my Church, my conscience, or your patient. I prayed, just as you might do, and I commended the soul of our brother to God. That's all: no more."

I knew it could not have been easy for a man of Father Liever's background and Order to act as he did that night. I had kept my promise to Peter Drasny, but Father Liever, by his breadth of understanding, had shown true Christianity, and had given one poor woman lifelong peace of mind.

But Fate had played a cruel game with her son.

Chapter
Thirty-three

"There's time for one more trip before the snow," said Alan Murray one evening. "Let's go riding."

We were sitting in Alan's house having a beer. There was Alan, myself and Howard Steele. Howard is a rancher from Turner Valley, about twenty-five miles west of Okotoks. It would be difficult to think of him as anything other than a rancher, with his blue jeans, buckskin jacket and well worn stetson, and on horseback he appears to be clamped to the saddle.

Alan Murray is a stocky, resilient fellow. As a part-time guide he has led geological exploration parties into forests or over mountain paths, using packhorses to carry supplies and equipment. He once said of such expeditions in "the old days" when helicopters were unknown, "You could be gone for weeks and when you got out of the mountains you didn't know till you phoned home whether your family was alive or dead."

The two are old friends. The story is told of them going off on a hunting expedition. Like careful men, they left word of their approximate whereabouts, but when they didn't return by the appointed time, a search party set out.

The hunting season is always a time for trouble. Inexperienced hunters are a menace, accidentally shooting themselves or other people. Ill-clad and not equipped to cope with the winter cold, without compasses or matches to light a fire, they can lose themselves and have to be rescued, sometimes minus a toe or two from the combined effects of inadequate footwear and frost-bite.

And sometimes they don't come back at all. Though my two friends were experienced, to say the least, there are still those treacherous mountain paths where horses can fall with their riders. However, it soon became obvious to the rescue party that there had been a sudden snowfall, heavy enough to make riding slow and difficult, which could explain the non-return of the hunters.

When, from a high bluff, they saw a strange light in the sky, the party struggled toward it, entered a clearing in the woods, and there discovered my friends seated in front of a roaring campfire, the essence of comfort. They had built a lean-to shelter against the prevailing wind, then heaped evergreen branches against the framework on top of which snow was piled as further insulation. The ground around the campfire had been cleared. The horses stood nearby, as comfortable as their masters. The latter were reclining against their saddles, insulated from the ground by a carpet of evergreens, saddle blankets and sleeping bags. They were cooking steaks and dispensing the first aid kit to one another – the first aid kit, by tradition, being a bottle of rum.

"Come on in," cried Alan. "You guys are just in time to join the party. We heard you coming through the bush. What's brought you out here? I suppose some fool's gone and lost himself!"

As one rescuer later told me, "All that pair needed to complete their night out were the dancing girls!"

Although a rookie, I had learned a lot, and once or twice a year we'd "go riding". This meant spending several days in the mountains riding over narrow paths, along the shores of mountain lakes, sparkling blue yet icy cold; or across lush alpine meadows, unexpected Shangri-Las in hidden valleys. It meant riding up steep slopes forested with pine and aspen, the woods thinning out at the treeline where even the wiry mountain grass would be sparse, and the rock face show through. Higher still the shale would be loose and treacherous and here the wise horseman led his mount. Sometimes the peaks towered high above us, with overhanging cliffs from which enormous boulders had hurtled down over the centuries to lie scattered on the level ground.

Far above, an eagle might launch itself from its eyrie and circle effortlessly in the sky, majestic, watchful. Silently I would sit in the saddle letting my horse nibble at the grass while I looked around, awed by the immensity of it all. Then, reminded of Man's insignificance in the face of Nature, I would touch the reins and ride quietly away.

"What about it, doc?" said Alan. "Can you arrange to get a couple of days off next week?"

My memories of past expeditions were suddenly at an end. Alan's question had brought me back from my reverie to the reality of his sitting room, to the beer glass in my hand.

"Sure. I'll get one of the men at High River to deal with emergencies," I replied. "I'll be there."

"Right. How about going up Mist Mountain?" asked Howard. "And we should look at Rickett's Pass. A week today – would that suit you fellows?"

It was agreed upon. We would truck our horses in to Mist Creek, about sixty miles west of Okotoks, and ride from there. The creek, a mountain stream, runs past a flat, open piece of land surrounded by trees, beyond which the mountains rise, gently at first and thickly forested. We had been there before and knew the very bank against which we would back the truck, so that we could safely unload the horses. We knew where we would pitch our tents. We would leave Okotoks before dawn. With luck we should be at our campsite by breakfast time, reach the pass by early afternoon and be back in camp before nightfall.

The week passed quickly. The night before we left, the horses were corralled at Alan's field, the harness was checked and arrangements made for an early departure. I slept fitfully that night and was out of bed at the first subdued ring of the alarm. All was dark. Janet stirred, smiled sleepily and said,

"Have a good time. Just don't fall off your horse."

She was asleep before I could inform her that I could not fall off my horse. No Westerner has ever been known to fall off his

190

horse. He may be "thrown off" or "bucked off", but falling off
is an unknown phenomenon in Alberta.

When I reached Alan's place, the animals were moving restlessly about the corral, watching the activity around them, paw-
ing the ground in search of some unnoticed blade of grass,
resentful of this sudden change in their routine, and well aware
that work lay ahead.

Our horses were old friends. Once on the trail they seemed
to enjoy these outings as much as we did. They were good-
tempered creatures and what is all-important in the mountains
– sure-footed. But they had to be loaded, all three of them, on
to one truck and this is a situation that calls for recognition of
protocol, for once aboard there would be some shoving, whinnying and tossing of heads, but they would soon settle down,
accepting the inevitable, for in many respects horses are like
human beings. I have heard it said that all horses are stupid.
That's not true. Some are lazy and won't work unless they have
to, just like their masters. Most are self-centered, but some
strive for dominance over other horses, while some are placid,
even amiable and take pleasure in the company of human beings.
Then there are those insufferable creatures who, at the least
opportunity and with surreptitious deliberation, will kick your
shins, or take the seat out of your pants at one bite, but many,
I am quite convinced, love to be shown affection and respond
to it.

I had little time to philosophize, however, as we loaded the
truck and saw the animals settled down. There were to be six
of us on this trip; our companions, Hugh and Mary Gillard and
Court Aggett, were expert riders. They arrived in their own
truck as we finished loading and we drove off in the two trucks
just before dawn.

Before us lay the foothills and behind them, silhouetted against
the pre-dawn sky, the mountains, ridge after ridge, peak upon
peak. Like a great spine hundreds of miles deep and two thousand miles long, they stretch from Canada's Northland into the
Western United States.

Soon we were into the hill country where the ground is too
rocky, the frosts too early for wheat to survive. The road surface
here was of gravel, and in the still autumn morning, a long trail

191

of dust hung in the air behind our little convoy as we drove into the first range of the Rockies, and to our campground at Mist Creek.

The aspens had been touched by an early frost. Their foliage stood out in shades of red and gold against the dark green of the surrounding pine trees. The sun had not yet warmed the high land, and the breeze rustling the dry autumn leaves increased the chill of the morning air as we set out about our tasks.

A campfire was lit, coffee made, the horses unloaded and saddled, sandwiches quickly eaten round the fire which was then extinguished before we mounted our horses and rode towards the mountain trail. There was little talking as, riding in single file, we checked our saddles, girths and stirrups. Only the steady clip-clop of the horses' hooves and the creaking of saddle leather disturbed the silence. We climbed steadily, traversing clearings that showed distant valleys with jagged peaks towering above them. I broke the silence.

"Alan," I said to my friend, who was riding immediately in front of me, "what beautiful country to ride in – or hike in!" And as an afterthought, I added, "but by gum, I'd hate to meet a bear!"

Alan turned in his saddle and grinned at me,

"This is bear country, all right. But you don't want to worry too much about bear – at least about black bear. If one's on his own and hears you coming, the chances are you'll never even know he's there. He'll move into the woods. Your average black bear no more wants trouble than you do. Mind you, it's a different business if you come across a mother with cubs. That's dangerous. But a black bear will usually get out of your way."

"And," added Howard with a laugh, "if he won't, just kick him up the ass!"

"I think," said Hugh Gillard, joining in the conversation, "you'd better be sure the doc knows the difference between a black bear and a grizzly before you give him that kind of advice. If he kicks a grizzly up the ass he's in trouble!"

"He knows," Howard said. "All bears are dangerous but the grizzly can be deadly. He can outrun a horse over a couple of hundred yards. Did you know that? A grizzly can kill an elk – a big elk – with one blow. I wouldn't want to walk into one of those characters on a dark night."

"And, Hugh," I concluded, "nothing in this world would tempt me to kick even the smallest bear up anywhere."

"Well," said Hugh, "it's not impossible. I know, because my Uncle Arthur did just that one night. Uncle Arthur used to live near Jasper and after my aunt died he just kept on a-going. His one pleasure was spending Saturday evenings at the hotel. He'd go and have dinner, then stay in the pub yarning till closing time.

"Anyway, late one Saturday night he got back to the house. He had to walk a bit to get to the door. He was almost up to the back door when he sees this black bear with its head right down inside the garbage can. It was one of those big galvanized garbage cans and the bear's hind legs were off the ground, he'd got so far in. He'd tilted the can towards him a bit.

"Uncle Arthur was an Englishman – you know the kind I mean," said Hugh, nodding significantly. "He didn't give one goddam about anyone or anything. I suppose, too, he wasn't feeling any particular pain, it being Saturday night. Anyway, he walks a few steps back, takes off at a run and plants one hell of a kick on that bear's backside."

"What happened?" I asked in trepidation.

"Well," said Hugh, "old Arthur told me afterwards he could hear that garbage can clanging off trees for half a mile down the trail. Uncle Arthur," he added, quite unnecessarily, "was a bit of a character."

For a time there was silence. The trail was strewn with fallen trees and the horses stepped gingerly over them. Sometimes, they jumped over them, which is all right as long as there are no overhanging branches. Then the rider's reaction time had better be fast.

We had seen no sign of wildlife. This was not surprising, for we announced our presence by attaching bells to our horses' harness. Wild animals heard the tinkling of the bells, and knowing man's capacity for destructiveness, they stayed out of our way.

As we neared the higher slopes, the views became breathtaking. Valleys clothed in the vibrant colors of autumn stretched as far as we could see, one merging with another, the rivers far below us irregular, silver threads. Alan, Howard and I were

193

riding together. Our companions had gone off on some exploration of their own, having arranged to meet us that evening at our camp.

It had been an enjoyable morning and I was relaxed – too relaxed. We were on a narrow, rocky path climbing a gorge. To our left and within reach was the rock wall. To our right was a steep, rocky slope, treeless and almost sheer for perhaps a hundred feet. Alan was riding immediately ahead of me. The horses were slowly poking along. Carelessly, I allowed mine to take his own pace, and before I realized what was happening he had decided to shove his nose at the rear end of the animal in front of him.

There was uproar. Alan's horse whinnied, bucked and lashed out with her rear hooves. My friend kept his seat and frantically I reined my animal back. It was over in a few seconds. No damage had been done, but it had been a lesson to me, and might have been an expensive one. I sometimes think that I keep getting lessons in this life and fail to profit by them, but this lesson's effect was permanent. I was never again a careless rider.

"Jeez," said Alan, with a wry grin, as he looked downwards, "I didn't much fancy going ass over tip down that." He followed that with a gem of advice.

"I tell you what, doc: there's only one golden rule about horses. If there's any trouble, I don't care how *nice* your critter is, that hoss won't give one goddam about you. Never forget that!"

The sun was at its height when we reached the treeline. The trees had become scarcer. Only pine and spruce could survive the winter cold at that height, but eventually even those began to thin out until we were riding in open country, the only vegetation scattered bushes and mountain grass.

Far above us we could see the summit of Mist Mountain, razor sharp against the blue sky. A mile or so away lay Rickett's Pass. The pass was a great cleft on the rock face, on the southern side of which began a narrow but passable path, leading to a small plateau and from there to the gentler slopes below. The

194

north slope was covered by loose shale and grass, but the southern exposure, warmed by the sun, was covered by grass and bushes.

Howard and I decided to ride on together. Alan wanted to explore a nearby valley to "case the joint" for a hunting trip later that fall, observing the numbers of elk, looking for vantage points and selecting a campsite. He rode off, disappearing into the trees.

We could see the pass now, a few hundred feet above us and perhaps half a mile away. The conformation of the ground had allowed a few trees to grow in sheltered places and we were emerging from one such glade when Howard suddenly reined in his horse.

"Look at that!" he exclaimed. "Something scared the daylights out of him!"

A big bull elk, magnificently antlered, galloped madly from the pass and raced onto the shale on the steep north slope. Small pieces of shale were thrown up around him like spray from a boat's bow as, with legs splayed out, he slid down the mountainside. Even when he reached flat ground his pace never slackened. He raced on like a mad thing and disappeared into the trees.

"My!" said Howard, reaching for his binoculars, "what a hurry to be in!"

He scanned the ground around the entrance to the pass, then handed the binoculars to me.

"Do you see anything move, doc?"

My search was equally unsuccessful.

"Well," said my companion, "we're going over there anyway, but we'll be careful."

A hundred yards from the summit Howard reined in his horse, dismounted and handed the reins to me.

"Keep the horses here. We don't want to get too close, for if they get a whiff of what I think is up there, they'll go like the wind for Okotoks; and it'd be a long walk home. I'll be back."

He was off, moving quietly from rock to rock, pausing occasionally to examine the terrain in front of him. I saw him get to within perhaps twenty yards of the pass, then he edged his way upwards, crawling for the last few yards before peering cautiously over the top. I could see him focus his binoculars, then settle down to watch something.

The horses were contentedly cropping the grass and I held the reins firmly, watching my friend, who after a time slipped backwards down the slope, turned and made his way to where I stood.

"Go and have a look," he said, "and take the glasses. You'll maybe never get a chance to see anything like that again. But go quietly."

I copied Howard's movements, reached the summit, slowly raised my head and looked over. Immediately I knew why the elk had panicked. Two hundred yards down the trail a huge silvertip grizzly was prowling around some bushes. I focused the glasses on him, very nearly followed the elk and might have outstripped him. The binoculars made the bear seem not two hundred yards away, but *two*. He was oblivious to any watcher and the wind, thankfully, was blowing my scent away from him.

The great silver-grey mane that gave him his name stretched down his back from the top of his massive head. He had a great paunch and probably was an old bear with his teeth bothering him, adding to his natural irritability, but I did not ponder that point. I was too busy being inconspicuous, but as the minutes passed, I became absorbed, then amused at his antics. He was enjoying himself! He would prowl around a bush, a great paw stretched out; tender branches were broken off and stuffed into his mouth. His lower jaw was stained purple from the berry juice. He was salivating and the saliva stained his beard. With the hump on his shoulders that proclaims the grizzly, the ponderous walk, the forward thrust of his heavy head, there was a terrifying impression of latent power. For a moment, and quite ridiculously, I thought of a film I had once seen of Sir Winston Churchill working in his garden at Chartwell!

Once he looked in my direction and momentarily panic-stricken though I was, I forced myself to "freeze", but he hadn't seen me and continued his perambulation of the bushes apparently in the best of good humor. Could this elderly gentleman, disporting himself so happily in his garden, I thought, really be *Ursus horribilis*, the Terror of the Rockies, the same animal that will kill black bears and eat them or his own young, for that matter? Surely not, I thought, as I watched him ponderously sit down. It would be falsifying fact to say that as he sat, he belched, but it is a pleasure to think that in his contentment, he may have done so. Then, ludicrously, he scratched his great paunch, lay back and rolled in the dust.

I looked back to where Howard stood with the horses. He waved to me to come back and so, reluctantly, yet more relieved than I cared to admit, I quietly returned to my friend.

"It'll begin to get dark soon," he said, "and we've got to get back before sunset."

It had been a memorable day. It was an equally memorable evening spent round the campfire, where we could dispense the first aid kit to one another, slide into our sleeping bags and fall asleep to the music of the mountains – the rustling of the leaves in the wind, the rushing and tumbling of the mountain stream, the far-off howling of coyotes.

Next day we struck camp and made for home. In the barbershop later that week, I talked about our trip, about our encounter with that magnificent old bear in Nature's garden. Word got around. Somebody went out to Mist Mountain, found our grizzly and for his hide to grace a floor, he shot him.

I know he was an old bear; his teeth perhaps were bothering him, and maybe he didn't have long to go, but I've often thought of Florence Freedman's poem –

> There were but two beneath the sky –
> The thing I came to kill, and I.
> I, under covert, quietly
> Watched him sense eternity,
> From quivering brush to pointed nose –
> My gun to shoulder level rose,
> And then I felt (I could not see)
> Far off, a Hunter watching me.
> I slowly put my rifle by,
> For there were two who had to die –
> The thing I wished to kill,
> And I.

197

Chapter
Thirty-four

"Could I just trouble you for some advice?" asked Mrs. Rootes when I picked up the telephone in answer to its ring. "I just hate to do this, for I know it must be nearly suppertime, but I'm a bit worried about Glen."

Glen was her husband, a sturdy, cheerful farmer, a man in his early forties, and not one given to being ill. The chances were that if Mrs. Rootes was worried, she had cause to be, and I placated her.

"He's not well," she said. "He's not been well for about two days. It all began with a sore throat, but he's just crawling about his work now. It's not like him at all, but he won't complain. What do you think I should do?"

"Sore throats are seldom things to get alarmed about," I said, "but how sick is Glen?"

"He looks rotten," replied his wife, "but I guess if you think it's nothing . . ." her voice trailed off.

"I didn't say that," I replied. "I just said that sore throats are seldom emergencies. And if there's one chap I know who wouldn't give in to any trifle, it's your better half. Look – I'm going to the hospital after supper and it'll hold me up by only about ten minutes to come round your way. I'll look in."

I put the phone down, had supper and drove to the hospital via the Rootes' place. They were the kind of people it was a pleasure to care for, and having turned aside offers of tea or coffee, I turned to my patient. His wife was right. He did look rotten. His normally ruddy complexion was a pasty grey. When I stepped into the living room he was lying on the couch, but made a half-hearted attempt to rise when he saw me.

"You're not looking your best, Glen," I said, smiling. "Let's have a look at this throat."

Almost casually I shone my flashlight down his pharynx and examined it. He had tonsilitis. There were the usual septic spots on his tonsils, both of which were inflamed and enlarged. His temperature was slightly raised. The diagnosis was easy to make, and as I had said earlier, hardly any emergency. Still, the Rootes were nice folk and I didn't make a fuss.

"Doc," said Glen, "could I have stomach flu with the tonsilitis?"

"Stomach flu?"

"Yes. I've had this pain in my stomach for a day or two now. My throat was so sore that my stomach seemed nothing. Now it's the other way round. I'm walking about half doubled up."

That was a different story, and not at all casually I examined Glen Rootes' abdomen. Low on the right side there was tenderness to touch. He flinched as I palpated the abdomen even gently. There was a lump there, not a very big lump perhaps, but enough to alert me to several ominous possibilities. He might have tonsilitis, but that was not the whole story.

"How long have you had this pain?"

"Two – three days, doc. It wasn't much to begin with."

"Well," I said, "there's one thing to be done, and that's have you in hospital. I don't know what this is. I can think of a number of things, but you must come into hospital for observation."

When we reached the hospital I called one of my colleagues into consultation. He was not at all happy with what he saw and suggested that we call Dr. Sinclair and ask him to see Rootes. Dr. Sinclair, another Scottish emigrant and a consultant in surgery, came at once from Calgary.

He was not only an excellent surgeon but a precise diagnostician, with a mind like a computer, I used to think. Unlike a computer, however, he also had the gift of clinical instinct. He had been a tutor in surgery at one of Britain's universities and his visits always became tutorial lectures that absorbed and enlightened us. He would discuss the X-ray and laboratory tests. Turning to the blackboard he would catalogue the diagnostic possibilities in a case, list the patient's symptoms and signs, then "work through the differential diagnosis" as he put it, until he had pinpointed the final diagnosis.

The surgeon came to the conclusion that Glen Rootes had an abscess around the appendix. He had probably, he said, had an appendicitis, an abscess had formed, and this had leaked slowly into the abdomen. Nature's defence, the omentum, a curtain-like membrane in the abdominal cavity, had had time to wrap

199

itself around the abscess which had been sealed off by the time I had seen the patient that evening.

"It's a very atypical appendicitis," I remarked, "no vomiting – insidious onset."

"That's often the case in middle-aged men," replied our surgeon, "and don't forget his tonsilitis either. There could easily be an association there."

That night I could see that he was having some difficulty in deciding whether or not he should operate.

"There's a very good chance," he told us, "that this abscess has sealed itself off. It's very localized and I'd rather choose my time to operate than treat the case as an emergency, open him up and maybe spread the abscess into his peritoneum. Besides, I want him to be given large doses of antibiotics before we do anything. And he needs fluid intravenously. He's already dehydrated."

It was decided that Rootes was to be watched very carefully. Blood tests to determine his bodily response to infection were taken every few hours and the pelvic lump was measured and "mapped out" in blue pencil on his abdomen, a little procedure that Glen Rootes greeted with wan amusement.

He seemed to improve overnight and when Dr. Sinclair came from Calgary in the morning, it was decided to watch our patient for another day. But that was not to be. Later in the afternoon he complained of increasing discomfort low in the abdomen. Blood tests indicated that the infection was not under control and the surgeon was informed.

"Get the operating room ready," was his laconic response to my telephone call. "I'll be down in an hour."

The operation was deftly done. Sinclair was an expert; I acted as the assistant surgeon. When the abdomen was opened, exposing the abscess surrounded by the omentum, he merely whistled, grunted, "What a shocker," and impassively set about his task.

Only the stump of the appendix was found but a large abscess cavity was opened, emptied, and a rubber drain left in. Sinclair handled the bowel with great gentleness, but it was a difficult surgical feat, even for him. Still, eventually it was done, and the surgeon departed, having given us his post-operative orders, and saying he would return the following morning.

Glen Rootes seemed to get almost immediate relief and greeted me in the morning with a smile. Sinclair saw him an hour or two later, expressed cautious satisfaction with the patient's condition, and left for Calgary.

It was two days later that our patient developed the first, ominous signs of paralysis of the bowel. His abdomen swelled to an alarming extent. The sounds of a normal bowel at work vanished. Even with the stethoscope I failed to find a murmur. Air was gathering in the intestine and soon Rootes' abdomen was like a huge football, hard and exquisitely tender to the touch.

Paralytic ileus of the bowel is relatively uncommon, can be caused by a number of conditions, and usually it can be dealt with.

Nowadays, it rarely kills. Glen Rootes, with his abscess, bowel inflammation and surgery on top of it all, had ample cause for this serious complication.

Drugs, intravenous fluids were given; tubes were passed to help the bowel gases to escape, but all to no avail. Dr. Sinclair visited every day, and I haunted the hospital morning and night, for we had no resident doctors to do routine work, or deal with emergencies. Then one morning the surgeon confirmed my growing and miserable fears.

"We're doing everything that can be done," he said. "He's going downhill, and he can't go on for long. He's either going to make it, or he's going to die, I'm afraid."

His care and concern had been exceptional and he was grim-faced as he made this forecast. When he left, I went back to see my patient. His face, sharp with pain and shock, was clammy and his eyes had the desperate look of a man fighting to survive.

"If I could just get some rest, doc," he half whispered. "I'm beat for sleep."

"We're trying everything, Glen," I replied. "You'll be all right," but I knew he didn't believe me, and disconsolately I walked along the corridor.

At the nurses' station I met my wife and Judy Sedgeley, the senior nurse. They were deep in conversation. Miss Sedgeley was already a very experienced nurse. She had been in charge of Glen Rootes from the beginning and had no illusions about what the future held for him. Nor had Janet, who had examined the man each morning with me.

They beckoned to me.

"What's the latest word on Mr. Rootes?" they asked.

"It couldn't be worse."

"We think," said Janet, "that you must hypnotize him."

"He's got a paralysis of his bowel," I replied. "Hypnosis isn't going to do a scrap of good in such a desperate situation. What's the point of even thinking about it?"

"We've been discussing the case," said Miss Sedgeley. "Despite all the drugs, he hasn't closed his eyes since the ileus began."

Said Janet, "If, by hypnosis, you could even produce some relaxation, it might help. I know it's not a scientific approach, but at this stage anything that might help is worth a try."

Thoughtfully I went back to Glen's room. I began,

"Glen, somehow we've got to get you some rest. I would like to use hypnosis. Are you willing to have a go?"

"I'll try anything," was the almost whispered response.

I began to lead him into a hypnotic trance. To my astonishment, he responded. His breathing deepened, his eyes closed and his arms relaxed, dropping limply to his sides. I told him that under hypnosis he would sleep until two o'clock that afternoon; that he would then waken refreshed. When I left he appeared, to the superficial observer, to be deeply asleep for the first time in days. I left orders that if there was any change for the worse I was to be notified at once. Otherwise he was to be watched carefully and the time that he wakened was to be noted.

Janet and I went back to Okotoks. In the middle of lunch the phone rang and an alarmed nurse told me that she had just checked Mr. Rootes.

"He's lying there with his mouth and eyes wide open. I can't rouse him. He seems to have gone into coma."

"Could I speak to Miss Sedgeley?"

"She's just left the floor for a moment. She's been with him all morning. I'll get her to phone you as soon as she returns."

"You haven't seen Mr. Rootes this morning?"

"No, I'm just keeping an eye on things for a moment. But he

looks dreadful and I've just read your orders that you were to be phoned . . ."

"Thank you. I'll come right up."

"Now," said Janet, "just hold on. Wait till Judy phones back. Remember you said he would sleep until two – he may be in a deep hypnotic state, not coma at all. And this nurse doesn't know the case."

In a few minutes we learned that not only had there been no deterioration in the patient's condition, but the rate and quality of his pulse had improved, though his abdomen remained grossly swollen.

At almost precisely two o'clock that afternoon he woke and said he felt quite a bit better. I visited him that night and although his abdomen was still distended, there was obvious improvement.

Janet and Judy were triumphant.

"See!" they cried, "there's something in your hypnosis after all." Still, I was skeptical and ill-at-ease. I slept badly that night and shortly after daybreak I drove to the hospital and headed for Glen Rootes' room. I met him in the corridor. Accompanied by a solicitous nurse, he was "going for a little walk," he said. His intravenous drip was still in place, suspended from a trolley the nurse was pushing in front of him.

I stopped in amazement.

"How d'ye feel, Glen?" I asked.

"Pretty good, doc, all things considered – especially since I had that sleep. But how do *you* feel? You look terrible!"

James Herriot, the world-famous author-vet, is an old friend of ours. Some years ago when Janet and I were visiting Yorkshire we renewed our friendship. One evening over dinner James and I reminisced about puzzling and interesting cases.

I told him about the strange recovery of Glen Rootes and I voiced my private doubts. Had "hypnotic sleep" really been the crucial factor in his survival that Janet and Judy Sedgeley believed it to be? Or had Glen's paralytic ileus simply reached a crisis in which he must either live or die?

"There are still so many mysteries in life," said Herriot, "in

203

your field and in mine. No doubt they'll mostly be explained one day."

I reminded him of the similarity of his own experience in a story he tells in *Vet in Harness*. He had been called out by a farmer. It was the lambing season, always a busy, worrying time for farmers and vets.

Herriot was confronted with the task of delivering a set of twins after the farmer's clumsy attempts at delivery had failed. Quite by accident, the vet discovered a second ewe lying neglected and in desperate straits in a dark corner of the stable. This one had lambed the previous day.

The farmer brusquely dismissed our friend's concern for the animal. It had had a "roughish time lambing," he said euphemistically. The animal was dying, he declared, and there was nothing Herriot could do for it.

That could be true, thought our friend, but when the farmer was busy elsewhere, he quietly gave the animal a large injection of Nembutal, a strong sedative.

"I made up my mind," he said reflectively, "that the poor creature wasn't going to suffer any more. If it had to die, at least it would die in peace."

But it didn't die and several days later when he paid another visit to the farm, an astounded Herriot was shown the ewe contentedly feeding in a field.

"That ewe just went to sleep," said its owner, blissfully unaware of our friend's attempt to ease the animal's "last" suffering. It had slept for two days. "And on t' third morning she was standing there lookin' at me and ready for some grub. Ah'll tell tha' young man, you'd just have thought she'd been drugged!"

Subsequently Herriot used induced sleep in another case – a dog this time, and again he found it to be excellent therapy. The dog recovered.

"So don't dismiss your experience too quickly," said our friend as he leaned over to refill my wine glass, "for it's amazing how all life has so much in common." He added with a smile, "To think that you made your little discovery on the Canadian prairies, and thousands of miles away I made mine on the floor of a dales stable! Wasn't it John Donne who said 'Sleep is pain's easiest salve'?"

Chapter
Thirty-five

Sleep!

> The death of each day's life, sore labour's bath,
> Balm of hurt minds, great nature's second course,
> Chief nourisher in life's feast.

Glen Rootes' health improved day by day. Whether the deep trance he experienced had anything to do with his dramatic improvement it is impossible to say. I can only speculate that hypnosis played a part.

Before I hypnotized him he appeared close to death, yet six hours later, after a profound "sleep", he declared he felt much better and attributed the change to rest – sleep. Although I had had extensive experience in the use of hypnosis, I was very skeptical of success when I began to induce the trance, regarding it as a forlorn and probably foredoomed attempt to help a gravely ill man. Today I cannot help feeling that there was more than coincidence involved.

I was not a novice. My interest in medical hypnosis had been stimulated more than ten years previously when I had watched a stage demonstration. Since then I had studied the subject, applied it in my practice, obtained the diploma of the American Board of Medical Hypnosis, become a member of the Society for Clinical Hypnosis, and later would lecture to physicians, psychiatrists and psychologists at university courses.

And yet, until recent years, hypnosis by and large was not recognized as a legitimate part of medical practice. True, there were experimental centers in some universities and research institutions, but the practising physician who spoke favorably about it, or admitted to using it in practice, was likely to be greeted by his colleagues with raised eyebrows or derisive smiles.

Hypnosis is a physiological state, sometimes resembling sleep, in which the hypnotized person shows an increased acceptance of suggestion. It has been defined too, as a state in which there is uncritical acceptance of suggestion. Hypnosis, in fact, can be defined fairly accurately in general terms. It can be described but it cannot as yet be explained. A great deal of what is written about it is speculation.

We have, all of us, experienced it at some time. It is a world-wide phenomenon, and probably as old as humanity itself. The steady lapping of waves on the seashore can induce a state of mind bordering on a trance. This is a mild form of self-hypnosis.

How many of us, when driving our cars, probably on a quiet sunny day, have wondered what happened to several miles of familiar highway that had passed unnoticed. That is mild self-hypnosis. At the least threat to safety we would, generally speaking, immediately have become alert.

The medical uses of hypnosis were known to the ancient priest-kings of Egypt, to the Druids of ancient Britain, and to the Chinese many centuries ago. In more modern times, the subject intrigued clinicians in Europe; notable among these was Franz Anton Mesmer who died in 1815. Mesmer was a brilliant Viennese physician. Hypnosis has sometimes been called Mesmerism, after him, but ironically it was Mesmer who cast hypnosis into the ill repute from which it would not recover for over a century.

When practising in Paris, where he became a fashionable and successful physician, Mesmer enshrouded his clinical practices in mystery. He was something of a showman. Showmanship has always been anathema to a group as jealous of its reputation for integrity as the medical profession, and a committee of inquiry into Mesmer's methods was convened. Among its distinguished members was Benjamin Franklin. Brilliantly, they missed the point. Mesmer's successes, they said, were merely the result of suggestion! Mesmerism was officially cast into the abyss of disrespect.

But there remained the adamant believers. James Esdaile, a Scottish surgeon practising in India in the middle of the nineteenth century, having watched fakirs perform hypnotic feats, saw the possibilities of using it as an anesthetic. He performed several thousand minor and over three hundred major operations using hypnosis as the only anesthetic. His operations, witnessed by British officers, were notable for their low post-operative death rate at a time when surgery was often a death warrant. His work was discredited by his colleagues in Scotland.

However, pioneers like Elliotson (professor of Medicine at the University of London), Braid (another Scottish surgeon), Bernheim, Coué, Charcot and Freud struggled on. Today hypnosis is once again a respected part of the practice of medicine and research workers throughout the world are struggling to unravel its mysteries.

Its mysteries have given it great public appeal. It is a fascinating subject for many people. Others, even scientists, still regard hypnosis with suspicion, for Mesmer's ghost, like Hamlet's, is still there in the background.

The clinical effects of hypnosis cannot be measured scientifically. It is a nebulous skill, part more of the art than the science of medicine, and today medicine is so scientific that we are in danger of ignoring what used to be called the art of practice.

Hamlet, after seeing his father's ghost, said,

"There are more things in Heaven and earth, Horatio,
Than are dreamt of in your philosophy."

I sometimes think that in this scientific age those words should be inscribed in stone over the entrance to every university, for we so often insist on "statistical evidence" or "concrete fact" before declaring some subjects valid objects for study. Philosophy should be the handmaiden of science. Pasteur, after all, had no "statistical evidence" that certain bacteria existed, but Pasteur probably knew his Shakespeare!

Just a decade or so ago, it was almost scientific heresy to suggest that the brain, or specific parts of the brain, might secrete drugs. The brain just didn't do such things, you'd often have been told.

But men and women of vision did not accept that dictum and we now know that the brain does indeed secrete drugs, the endorphins. And we know that the endorphins are more potent than morphine. What we don't as yet know is how they are activated. We know very little about the human mind. And the human mind is one of the great, undiscovered frontiers of Medicine.

I had no lofty philosophical thoughts running through *my* mind when Tommy Denton caught up with me in the Okotoks main street. I had just finished a morning session in the office and my thoughts didn't extend further than my lunch.

Tommy was rather a favorite of mine. He was a bright, friendly little urchin of about ten years of age.

"Please, Doctor Gibson," he said, tugging at my sleeve. "Can I have ten cents?"

I regarded Tommy with assumed outrage.

"Tommy," I said severely, in my broadest accent, "that's an awful lot of money," but I ferreted in my pocket and produced a dime.

"Not *that* one!" said Tommy indignantly. "The one you owe me. The one you put on top of the towel rack!"

And then I remembered. Several weeks before, Mrs. Denton had brought Tommy to see me. His hands were covered in warts. They coalesced into a mass of excrescences on the poor youngster's hands. I tried all the recommended remedies – none of them worked. The warts continued to spread. Then, in a British journal, I read an article on folk medicine. A particular old lady, it was reported, could cure warts by rubbing a raw onion over them, then burying the onion under an oak tree at the full of the moon.

That was going a bit too far, I thought. Besides, there weren't any oak trees around Okotoks. Perhaps a cottonwood tree might suffice, I thought, but in the next issue, a chap said he knew of another remedy for warts. He knew of an old man who bought them.

My Scottish blood warmed to that. I'd rather have sold them, of course, but on Tommy's next visit, I bought his warts. I treated him first to a hypnotic TV show.

"Tommy," I said, as he sat in the office chair, "see that panel on the wall over there? What's your favorite TV show?"

"Buck Rogers."

"OK. When you're ready, you're going to see the best Buck Rogers show you've ever seen."

I led him into a trance and watched my young friend twitch his way through a show he later told me was "just great." During the show I told him I intended to buy his warts from him. They would be gone in a week, I said, and at the end of the show he solemnly watched as I put a ten cent piece on top of the towel rack.

It was a week later. There he stood before me in the sunlit Okotoks main street, his hands extended for my inspection.

The warts had vanished. He accompanied me to the office. Solemnly he watched as I retrieved the dime from the towel rack and handed it to him.

My purchase had been a bargain on both sides.

Chapter
Thirty-six

"Why is it," asked my charming hostess, "that medical schools are the only institutions of higher learning that give diplomas in omniscience?"

Janet and I were in Seattle, where I had been asked to lecture on medical services. It was a cruel thrust, coming from such a charmer – at a cocktail party too – and delivered with deadly sweetness. Of course I later had Janet's equally honeyed assurance that such a rapier-like remark could not possibly have been meant for me, but all the same I have often thought of my hostess' words, applied of course, to other members of my profession.

There is this story about the famous physician who died and went to heaven. He was so very famous that St. Peter, who met him at the heavenly gates, told him he had been asked to show him around. As they strolled along, the great physician was astounded to come upon a group of angels, standing in line, bosoms bared, their wings trailing in the celestial clouds, waiting to be examined by a benevolent looking elderly gentleman, who, stethoscope in place, was listening to heart sounds.

The famous physician stopped in his tracks.

"St. Peter," he cried, "I had no idea that you would require doctors in heaven."

"We don't," replied the archangel, "and lower your voice, sir; that's not a doctor. That's God. He likes to play doctor."

I have met doctors who play God; not many, but the omniscient are always among us. The vast majority of us have learned some hard lessons along the way and our feet are planted firmly on the ground – most of the time.

Then at a slightly lower level of command, there are those who practise messianic medicine, totally convinced that they, and they alone, can give the correct advice or do some operation most successfully, however much some other doctor should be consulted for the patient's safety.

I believe I can claim with reasonable honesty that in my work I have tried not to appear to be omniscient. Sometimes, on the other hand, an appearance of omniscience is not only required, it is expected. And on occasion it can be psychologically sound and desirable.

In Okotoks I used to keep two books on my desk top. They were both fairly heavy volumes. One, *French's Index of Differential Diagnosis*, was my diagnostic Bible. The other was a readable, concise textbook of medicine. I kept them on the desk top rather than on the bookshelf behind me because I consulted them so often.

One day, however, a patient seeking advice about some obscure symptoms, looked at me askance when I reached across the desk and opened *French's*.

"Do you need to look at that book?" he asked. "Don't you know what's wrong without having to read to find out?"

His tone of voice conveyed a rebuke, a hint of lost confidence, and the totally unwarranted – and now shattered – belief that I should have been omniscient.

My profession still stands high in public regard. It was not always so, perhaps for the simple reason that at first, unscientific pills and potions were usually placebos and often didn't work. But about a century ago, science made its great entry into medicine, and it changed the whole status of my profession. Doctors gradually achieved public esteem, and often a popular reputation for omniscience. Sometimes they were looked up to

210

as men learned in all aspects of the human condition, and the giants among them were all of that.

Some years ago I attended a medical conference in London. There was a session on "dealing with patients" to which medical students and teachers of medicine were invited. I was then a country doctor in Okotoks, but was also a part-time teacher in the department of family medicine at the University of Calgary Medical School, so I decided I should attend.

It turned out to be a dull affair. It was a delightful day outside; one of those warm hazy days that can make London a joy for the visitor and my thoughts and eyes began to wander. The speaker, too, was wandering. He was talking about the "potentially antagonistic and inhibitory relationship between prescribing physician and the non-compliant patient relative to the totality of ingested medication" – in other words, dealing with folks who wouldn't take their medicine.

I could be excused, I'm sure, for looking out of the lecture room window at Regent's Park at its best. However, things improved when a medical student from one of London's sainted hospitals rose languidly to his feet.

"I have simply no difficulty in dealing with patients," he drawled. "I merely imitate my betters and behave like God."

"Now there," I said to my companion, a New York surgeon, "is a chap with a sense of humor."

I knew exactly what the student meant. That morning I had strolled along nearby Harley St. and had actually seen a god descend from his Rolls Royce and enter his consulting rooms, there to deliver judgment. There was no doubt about it. His demeanor was that of a god, just like some of the gods I had known when I was a medical student. I smiled at the young man's quip, but horror overcame amusement when I realized he was in deadly earnest.

There are several saintly hospitals in London. They are deservedly world famous. Saint Bartholomew's is one, and is "Bart's" to its denizens, while Saint Thomas's (or Thomas's) is another. Depending on which side you are on, you can say, "you can always tell a Thomas's (or a Bart's) man – but you can't tell him much" and that student's remark gave me some of the answer to that jibe, for attitudes are passed on and perpetuate themselves. On the other hand, some of the most famous physicians I have met have been humble, open-minded men.

Sometimes, however, it is necessary or advisable to play God. It may serve a purpose where a patient is apprehensive and may do some temporary good, but it isn't an attitude that one should embark on lightly.

Othello believed in a cruel God, and I have known god-physicians (but thankfully, rarely) to be cruel.

A friend of mine, a competent and caring family doctor, discovered some suspiciously enlarged glands in a patient's neck. He referred his patient to a specialist.

"I sent him to that specialist," he later told me in tones of outrage, "because I was told he was good."

The specialist may have been "good" in a technical sense, but a few days later he phoned the patient direct. "Mr. Jones," he said without preamble. "The tests are back. You've got cancer. If I were you, I'd put your affairs in order. You don't have long to go."

He might have been telling that devastated man that he didn't need to bother about next week's groceries.

He had played God, making the ultimate judgment: the cruel, utter denial of hope. So, even if we doctors sometimes feel it necessary to be god-physicians, it is essential that we show compassion; otherwise, we fail both as doctors and as human beings.

I can only describe Margaret Boston as an irreverent patient. She would insist on questioning my reasons for doing this or that, but the grin that appeared so easily on her pleasantly attractive face made her a welcome visitor to the office.

Not that visits to the office were commonplace. The Bostons were sturdy, independent farmers and took care of most of their medical problems quite capably without my help. But when Margaret arrived in my sanctum one day, sat down and said,

"I'm sick, sick, sick," I knew I faced a challenge.

"Well," I remarked in my best professional manner, "we'll have to find out what's causing this."

Mrs. Boston looked at me.

212

"I can tell you what's causing it," she said. "It's simple. I'm pregnant. But I just can't stop this vomiting. I throw up from morning till night."

"How far on are you?"

"About six weeks, so I don't suppose there's any point in examining me yet; but if you could do something to stop the vomiting I really would be grateful."

Suddenly I realized that her smile was a bit forced, that her cheerfulness hid her tiredness.

Nausea in early pregnancy is not unexpected, I told her, affecting maybe half of all pregnant women, and the vomiting that sometimes accompanies it is also common. Happily it clears up spontaneously about the third month. My patient nodded at my reassurance.

"I know," she said, "I've had it before, and it's always gone on its own, but this time it's really severe."

So I gave her a prescription for tablets and told her to take two of them each bedtime. Then I prescribed a suitable diet and told her I'd see her in a week if she was no better.

In a week, when she did return, the smile she gave me was wan. She was tired, sleeping badly and the vomiting was undiminished, so much so that I wondered if she might be progressing towards *hyperemesis gravidarum*, or pernicious vomiting, a sometimes serious complication of pregnancy requiring hospital treatment.

It is said that emotional factors can play a part in this condition, but I felt intuitively that such was not the case here, and when I raised the possibility, my patient smiled.

"You know better than that, doctor," she said. "That Dan of mine is one of the best. He's more worried than I am – and we've no other worries. It isn't that, and I'm not going into any hospital either. I'm needed out at that farm. So be a good guy and try something else."

I consulted the books on my desk, just to make sure I was on the right track. Mrs. Boston didn't mind my doing that and smiled when I told her how, a week or two before, I had been chided for "reading up" on some symptoms I couldn't understand.

"You just go straight ahead," she said. "Try anything you have to, but just don't put me in hospital – that's all I ask."

From one treatment I went to others, all unsuccessfully. I tried hypnosis, which had sometimes worked in preventing vomiting or nausea. Useless. I saw her every couple of days. I could see she was beginning to lose weight. My worry increased, and I suggested that she see a specialist.

"Not on your life," objected my patient. "You know what a specialist'll say: 'hospital for you, my girl'. No. I've licked this before and I'll lick it again. Just you keep on trying. Something'll do the trick."

I had exhausted my little list of drugs and didn't know where to turn for help, when one day a drug traveler came into the office. He was a nice chap; I'd known him for five years and he had always given me sound advice on the latest in medications. I was telling him about my problem with Mrs. Boston, when he raised his hand and interrupted me.

"I have the very thing," he told me. "It's very new. Guaranteed to work in almost any case of vomiting. Here's a packet of a dozen tablets. Just try them on your patient."

Gratefully I accepted them, and next day I gave them to Mrs. Boston.

"Try them," I said, "and let me see you in two days. If this doesn't work, you'll be a good lass, won't you, and let me send you to a specialist? You just cannot go on like this."

She agreed. In two days she phoned me.

"I don't think I'll come in today. I really believe I'm feeling better."

This was good news and I told her that unless she had problems she should report for a routine physical examination in four weeks' time. The Margaret Boston that appeared four weeks later was her usual smiling, self-possessed self, and her pregnancy was advancing uneventfully.

One night, a month or so later, Janet and I were reading the latest medical journals.

"Listen to this," said my wife. "Here are reports of dreadful deformities occurring in the newborn, and studies that point to the use of a new drug. One I've never heard of."

"What's it called?"

214

"Thalidomide."

"I've never heard of it either," I said – and then suddenly I cried, "what's it called again?"

"Thalidomide. Apparently if taken in early pregnancy to counteract nausea, the number of cases of deformities in babies – no legs or arms – is simply horrendous."

"Oh! my God," I said despairingly, "that's the stuff I gave to Margaret Boston."

We pored over the article, the first to appear in Canada on the subject. The tragedy of thalidomide, and the awful deformities it caused, had just begun. The problem was first detected in Europe. According to the article, I had given my patient the pills at the very worst time, and in sufficient numbers to be catastrophic. Even a dozen pills could have a terrible effect.

Aghast, I stared at my wife.

"Her chances of having a deformed child are about ninety percent," I said. "What can we do?"

"What's done, is done," said Janet, who is a very rational person, "and cannot be undone. You'll have to tell her."

Mrs. Boston was by now six months advanced in pregnancy.

"No," I replied. "Not yet, anyway. There's a chance that she'll be one of the lucky ones. I'll tell her nearer the time."

We debated the matter. My firm viewpoint carried the day and three months of purgatory began for me.

I liked Margaret Boston and her husband. They were genuine, friendly folk. They had put their trust in me. I dreaded to think of what was going on in her womb, and could hardly face her when, so cheerfully, she came for her monthly pre-natal examinations. My blunder followed me on our summer holidays. I couldn't sleep. We were in a motel in California on our holiday when, in the middle of the night, Janet and I had a heated argument as to the proper course to take. My summer was ruined.

"It's done. What will be, will be. You weren't to know," Janet said. "Nobody knew what those pills could do. But you *must* tell her when we get home."

"I'll speak to her husband when we get back."

"All right, but I think you should tell Margaret."

"I'll speak to Dan."

215

When we returned to Okotoks, miserably I sought out Dan Boston and told him the story. He listened, poker-faced, then said,

"What are Margaret's chances of having a deformed baby?"

"Ninety percent."

To my amazement, Dan Boston tried to comfort *me*.

"It can't be helped, doc. It wasn't your fault. We'll just have to hope. There's no point in worrying Margaret. You and I will keep this to ourselves."

Margaret's baby was due in a few weeks. Margaret was the picture of health, but I made some excuse and sent her to a firm of specialists in X-ray work. I wrote to them:

"This lady was given twelve tablets of thalidomide in the first trimester of pregnancy. I greatly fear that her baby will be deformed. After X-raying her, could you let me have your findings?"

The report arrived within a few days.

"Your suspicions," they said, "appear to be justified. We cannot completely visualize the right leg; in particular the fibula and tibia of the lower leg are not visualized. The left arm appears to be foreshortened. The findings are compatible with thalidomide intake."

Wordlessly I handed the report to Janet.

"Now," she said, "you *must* tell that woman."

I nodded. "I'll be seeing her in a few days. Then I'll tell her."

But those few days never arrived. Margaret Boston went into labor. Usually I loved delivering babies, but I dragged myself to the hospital for this one.

It was Margaret's third baby. I warned the nurse, an old friend, of my fears. There was no point now, at this stage, in warning the mother, I thought, since the labor was obviously going to be a short one. The delivery progressed quickly, but it was with a heavy heart and leaden hands that I eased the baby into the world.

It was a little beauty, all pink and quivering and surprised; with two blue eyes and two podgy little legs and two podgy, perfect little arms and ten toes and ten fingers.

Seldom have I experienced greater relief or joy than at that moment. Still – there was the heart: that could be deformed.

216

No Swiss watch ever ticked more sweetly than little Miss Boston's heart. But before I'd let her mother touch her, I went over the baby with a fine toothcomb.

She was perfect.

Then I went to see Dan, anxiously waiting for me in a side room. He was sitting there, suddenly old-looking and tired, restlessly turning the brim of his hat between his hands. Shoulders hunched, he was watching the door as I came in, still in my hospital "greens" and gown. He started up when he saw me. My face proclaimed my message. He almost ran to meet me.

"Doc," he burst out. "It's all right, eh? It's all right?"

"Thank God, Dan – it's a perfect little girl."

We shook hands, laughed with relief and he said,

"You were so sure there'd be something wrong. How come, d'you think there wasn't?"

"Luck. Just luck, Dan."

"Can I go see her?"

"You can see them both. They'll be in the ward by now."

High River Hospital is a comfortable place, and a warm place, justly proud of its good name, and I knew that my patient would by now be in the brightly curtained, comfortable maternity ward, with its intimacy, its two patients to a room, their needs attended to by efficient, pleasant nurses.

With a wave, "father" was off, and equally quickly I was on my way down that little highway to Okotoks to tell Janet the good news.

All went well, and mother and baby were discharged from hospital, with instructions to see me in our Okotoks office in ten days' time. When they came in, Margaret Boston lovingly held her daughter out for my inspection.

But I still had suspicions. I wanted to be sure.

"Margaret," I said, "I'm going to examine this little thing again, if you don't mind."

"I don't mind."

So I examined the baby all over again, looking everywhere I could think of, feeling limbs, testing movements, looking in eyes, listening to its little heart. It was a pretty thorough "going over" and Mrs. Boston watched my every move.

217

Nothing. A normal infant, bright, alert, faultless. When I finished, a thoughtful-looking mother dressed her baby, then turned to me.

"That was quite an examination! So was the one you gave her when you delivered her. What's it all been in aid of?"

"Well, I just like to be thorough, you know."

"Not this thorough. Besides, you've not been yourself with me these last two months. I can tell. You were a bit strange. You had something on your mind. Now what was it?"

So I told her. I told her how as a last resort, I had given her twelve tablets of thalidomide – the last tablets I had tried. Of course the thalidomide tragedy was now at its height and the newspapers were full of it.

"Why didn't you tell *me*?"

"For your own sake, my dear."

"Did you tell anybody else?"

"Dr. Janet."

"Well, I'm sure you did. Did you tell anybody else?"

While I hesitated she said, "You see, another guy who was a bit strange recently is my husband. Did you tell him too?"

"Yes," I confessed. "I did."

"So you two were in cahoots with one another, trying to protect a poor, weak woman? And both of you worried to death, I suppose?"

"Well, you could put it that way," I said awkwardly. I didn't enlarge on my private purgatory of that summer.

Mrs. Boston suddenly burst into laughter – peal after peal of laughter. I couldn't stop her. It was acute, delayed hysteria, of course, immediately and easily diagnosed. I tried to calm her and eventually succeeded.

"Oh dear," she said, finally recovering her breath. "But I could have saved you two fellas an awful lot of trouble."

"What d'ye mean?"

"Those last pills? – I never touched them! They're still in the medicine cabinet. You can have them back anytime. The vomiting just cleared up by itself." And off she went again, into gales of laughter.

"When I think of you two guys keeping it all to yourselves . . ." she gasped. "Men . . ." she went on.

218

I found it difficult to join in her mirth. I had spent a considerable amount of money in going to California, and it had been wasted. No Scot likes to see money thrown away.

But I learned something from that case. I added another book to the two already on my desk – a book on the properties and clinical uses of drugs. And I never again put any ideas into the heads of any specialist in radiology, however eminent. The power of suggestion can affect even the mighty.

And I never again played God.

Chapter
Thirty-seven

Our decision to emigrate had not been easy. We were approaching middle age and we were very British. We were not carefree young adventurers who could view the whole thing as an exciting interlude before settling down to steady work. Above all, Catriona's future was of immense importance to us, and yet we had burned our bridges behind us – leaving friends we loved and a country we admired, because of the conditions of work there.

And yet, I sometimes wonder if there was not some deep-seated compulsion about it too. The Scots have always been emigrants. It is a tradition. Did the frustrations of working under the National Health Service merely bring some subconscious urge in me to the surface?

Janet and I both had difficulties to overcome and yet, as she wrote to our friends, the Herriots, in Yorkshire a few months after we arrived, how could we feel we were in a foreign country? Calgary's mayor was one Donald MacKay and the militia regiment was the Calgary Highlanders. We had Lord Strathcona's Horse, the MacLeod Trail, Burns' Trail and the nearby towns of Cochrane, Airdrie and Fort MacLeod.

Although many years have passed since that lonely day when the taxi driver dumped our flight bags on the dusty roadway outside the Willingdon Hotel in Okotoks and said, "You're home," I've never forgotten it.

Home! I can still see the wooden false-fronted shops and the graveled road. As that cab turned and headed back to Calgary I felt I had severed the last links to a life that was behind us forever. Since then dozens of friends have told me how they shared that feeling as they disembarked with their families at St. John's, Newfoundland, Auckland, New Zealand, or Sydney, Australia. Most of us, I think, found fulfilment. A whole new world of medicine opened for me.

We came to a part of Canada that was proud of its British heritage. It took us two years to establish our practice and we might have left, like the doctors who preceded us, but we were determined to serve a community that needed us rather than go to some city practice. It was very difficult at that time to attract doctors to small towns with limited facilities when the cities were growing rapidly and developing excellent medical facilities.

The Chamber of Commerce had brought us to Okotoks, but it was the Town Council that established us there.

One afternoon a few weeks after we arrived in Okotoks, we were told that a "town picnic" was to be held in the public park that evening. It would be nice if we could attend, we were told. Unsuspecting and rather shyly, Catriona, Janet and I walked to the park. There was a huge bonfire burning near the riverside. It was our first experience of a wiener roast. Trucks and cars kept arriving, their stetson-hatted owners gathering around the fire talking to one another, exchanging the agricultural gossip of the day.

Then they began to talk to us, introducing themselves, bidding us welcome.

There must have been two or three hundred people there when George Locke, the mayor, a clean-cut, articulate chap of about my own age, climbed on to a truck and called for silence.

"You all know why we're here," he said. "We're here to welcome our new doctors, the Gibsons, and their daughter Catriona to Okotoks."

There was a polite clapping of hands and some nodding of heads in our direction, as we stood there, embarrassed.

"There's more to it than that," exclaimed his worship. "You all know we haven't had a regular doctor since Dr. Ardiel died. We've had doctors in and out of this town for years now. Well, we think the Gibsons want to stay here. That depends on you. If you support them, the council is convinced they'll stay. It's not easy to attract doctors to small towns like this. You remember that. And remember, too," he finished, "we've not just got one doctor – we've got two, for the price of one!"

Sometimes at the beginning we were paid in eggs or sides of beef, but the "bad debts" we had been warned to expect never materialized.

We both had difficulties, of course. For one thing, we had to be careful about the idioms we used. I kept saying to patients as I gave injections, "this'll just take half a tick," to be met with blank looks at my use of this strange remark. On her part, Janet, until she learned the Canadian meaning of the remark, would keep encouraging men to "keep their pecker up," but on the whole we managed to adjust very nicely.

Janet managed to combine her role of mother and physician by arranging to hold her office sessions during school hours. However, when emergencies did occur and I was not available, people came to her. We furnished a small emergency office in the basement of our home where she could see such cases.

The nearest medical help was likely to be found at our door and people would sometimes drive there with very ill patients in their cars. If we were not around they'd carry on to the hospital.

We enjoyed the advantages of practice in a small community – the comradeship and close relationships that can develop between doctors and the families they serve. But we suffered from the disadvantages, too. We were constantly on call, and when we were out of town, tragedies sometimes occurred that might have been prevented had we been there.

I did most of the traveling and after a hard day's work, driving to the hospital a second time to meet patients there could be tiring as well as time-consuming. It was often just as easy to see them in their own homes or in our office in the town.

And there were the inevitable emergencies. I recall how one day, I was at the hospital when Janet received a call to an outlying farm. The farmer's wife had had a serious accident. She had been charged and butted by her pet cow, an animal she had raised from infancy. When she reached the farm gate, Janet found the farmer's son waiting for her. He was driving a tractor, the only vehicle that could negotiate the flood of water and mud from the spring run-off. Janet, clinging to the tractor driver, made it safely to her patient who had been dreadfully injured about the body, face and head.

Janet's examination revealed a broken jaw, fractured nose and a possible skull fracture plus numerous painful lacerations and bruises. After attending to her injuries and easing her pain, Janet made her patient as comfortable as possible in her own bed. Realizing that the flood water and muddy roads made transportation to the hospital impossible for her patient in her condition, she gave instructions for her care at home and made arrangements for her to be transported to hospital for X-rays as soon as conditions permitted it. Having done everything possible, she climbed back on the tractor for the return trip through the flood waters to the gate. She couldn't help thinking,

"Cripes, if my friends in England could only see me now!"

But Okotoks was not an isolated community. The city boundaries of Calgary were a mere twenty-five miles away, though in the depths of winter in a ditched or stalled car, one could feel utterly alone a few miles from home.

We joined the Calgary Philharmonic Society and drove regularly to the concerts. In winter people would look at us as we arrived in furs and snowboots and say,

"But surely you're not driving back *tonight!*"

But there was no danger to the drive if one was careful and watched the weather.

Within a few months of our arrival the last vestiges of homesickness had gone. We were living in a country where there was great openness, warmth and friendship. There was a tremendous feeling of drive and optimism, and I knew what old Mrs. Hogge meant when she said, "You've come to God's country".

Sometimes our intellectuals write despairingly of the Canadian identity. What is it? they will say. The lack of a Canadian identity worries them. Are Canadians merely colonial castaways of their mother countries: Frenchmen who speak an obsolete patois of old France; or Englishmen cast adrift by England; or Scots and Ukrainians, Danes and Dutchmen whose only common bond is their citizenship? And worst of all, some will say, aren't Canadians merely imitators of their cousins to the south?

Years after we became friends, Mrs. Hogge was invited to appear as a guest of honor at the Calgary Stampede. Janet and I watched as that slim, erect little figure was ushered on to the great open air stage. It was late evening. There were thousands of spectators in the grandstand and on the bleachers. Just in front of her was the racetrack with horsemen grouped around the stage.

Suddenly the spotlight was focused on her as the announcer who had ushered her on stage grasped the microphone.

"Ladies and gentlemen!"

There was a sudden hush.

"Ladies and gentlemen, I want to introduce to you Mrs. Catherine Hogge of Okotoks. She was the first white girl to come to this part of Alberta – in 1883. And she came all the way from Winnipeg by covered wagon. Give Mrs. Hogge a great hand."

The evening show wasn't over. The finals of the chuckwagon races were yet to come and the crowd was only mildly interested in one of Alberta's pioneers. There was polite handclapping. Mrs. Hogge was asked to say a few words.

"I should like you to know," she said, clearly and with great firmness, "that I did not come west by *covered wagon*. Americans came west by covered wagon. I came by Red River cart. *I* am a Canadian."

As one man, that enormous crowd rose to its feet and cheered her to the echo. Neither Mrs. Hogge nor her audience was having any trouble about identity!

And I was beginning to understand what was in Edward Chapman's heart when he wrote,

> Out where the hand clasp's a little stronger,
> Out where the smile lasts a little longer,
> That's where the West begins.